OCT 1 0 REC'D

D0044672

Mary Harper, Africa Editor, BBC World Service, author of *Getting Somalia Wrong?*

A meticulously detailed and empathetic work on a woman whose life should not be forgotten.

Richard Barrett, director of the Global Strategy Network and former director of global counter-terrorism at MI6

As well as telling a compelling story with great skill, this absorbing and clear-eyed examination of the work of one of East Africa's greatest humanitarians, based on her letters and interviews with her closest associates, also highlights the cultural challenges faced by even the most dedicated worker. Rachel Pieh Jones raises questions about motive and consequence, as well as perception and jealousy, that resonate well beyond the fascinating life she describes.

Mariam Mohamed, former First Lady of Somalia

Annalena Tonelli's story challenges readers to believe in themselves and reminds us that we can choose acts of kindness and love even during difficult circumstances. Her courage inspires us to challenge evil: everyone can make a difference.

Eboo Patel, founder and president, Interfaith Youth Core, author of *Acts of Faith*

My life has been shaped by the examples of faith heroes: Dorothy Day, Mahatma Gandhi, Martin Luther King Jr., Malcolm X. In this book, Rachel Pieh Jones introduces me to one more – Annalena Tonelli. Her example of immersive, selfless service combined with learning from different traditions should inspire us all.

Jason Fagone, author of *The Woman Who Smashed Codes*

A stunning meditation on love and service, this book has given me a new hero: Annalena Tonelli, a woman of faith who crashed through boundaries and dodged bullets in her mission to heal the sick. Author Rachel Pieh Jones has done justice to an extraordinary person, crafting a story every bit as vivid, relentless, and surprising as her subject.

Tom Krattenmaker, *USA Today* columnist, author of *Confessions of a Secular Jesus Follower*

Rachel Pieh Jones has given us the unforgettable story of a servant of the sick and poor who demonstrated, to an almost incomprehensible degree, what it means to love the least of these. Few of us will ever come close to Annalena Tonelli's devotion and bravery. But thanks to this remarkable book, we can be acquainted with one of history's great and unheralded exemplars, and inspired to give more of ourselves to those without.

Jordan Wylie, author of *Citadel* and *Running For My Life*

A fascinating, powerful, and extremely moving true story that needs to be shared with the rest of the world.

Stronger than Death

Stronger than Death

How Annalena Tonelli Defied Terror and Tuberculosis in the Horn of Africa

Rachel Pieh Jones

PLOUGH PUBLISHING HOUSE

Published by Plough Publishing House
Walden, New York
Robertsbridge, England
Elsmore, Australia
www.plough.com

Plough produces books, a quarterly magazine, and Plough.com to encourage people and help them put their faith into action. We believe Jesus can transform the world and that his teachings and example apply to all aspects of life. At the same time, we seek common ground with all people regardless of their creed. Plough is the publishing house of the Bruderhof, an international Christian community. The Bruderhof is a fellowship of families and singles practicing radical discipleship in the spirit of the first church in Jerusalem (Acts 2 and 4). Members devote their entire lives to serving God, one another, and their neighbors, renouncing private property and sharing everything. To learn more about the Bruderhof's faith, history, and daily life, see Bruderhof.com. (Views expressed by Plough authors are their own and do not necessarily reflect the position of the Bruderhof.)

ISBN: 978-0-87486-251-5

23 22 21 20 19   1 2 3 4 5 6 7 8

All cover images and photograph page 14 courtesy of the author. Photograph page 29 from Robert Estall Photo Agency / Alamy. Photograph page 119 from Agencja Fotograficzna Caro / Alamy. Photograph page 201 by Eric Lafforgue / Alamy.

A catalog record for this book is available from the British Library.
Library of Congress Cataloging-in-Publication Data

Names: Jones, Rachel Pieh, author.
Title: Stronger than death : how Annalena Tonelli defied terror and
   tuberculosis in the Horn of Africa / Rachel Pieh Jones.
Description: Walden, N.Y. : Plough Publishing House, 2019.
Identifiers: LCCN 2019017634 (print) | LCCN 2019018820 (ebook) | ISBN
   9780874862539 (Epub) | ISBN 9780874862515 (hardback)
Subjects: LCSH: Tonelli, Annalena, 1943-2003. | Lawyers--Italy--Biography. |
   Nurses--Africa, East--Biography. | Human rights workers--Africa,
   East--Biography. | Italians--Africa, East--Biography. |
   Tuberculosis--Hospitals--Somalia--Borama (Awdal)
Classification: LCC HV687.5.A353 (ebook) | LCC HV687.5.A353 J66 2019 (print)
   | DDC 362.109676--dc23
LC record available at https://lccn.loc.gov/2019017634

Printed in the United States of America

in memory of Anna Jewell
forever in our hearts

Contents

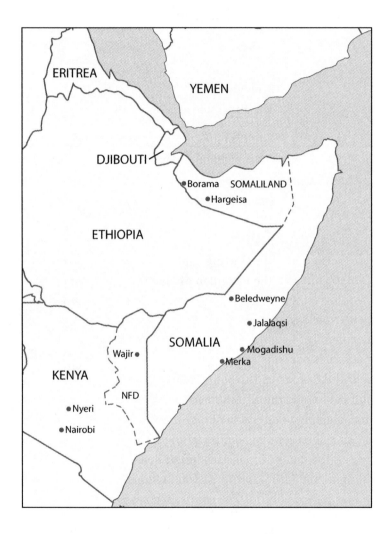

Prologue

ON OCTOBER 5, 2003, in a country that didn't exist, Annalena Tonelli performed routine checks on tuberculosis patients. They slept in huts in the courtyard of the Borama Tuberculosis Hospital and on cots in long rows inside sick wards. Annalena stopped at each hut, each bed. After sunset, darkness in the remote Somaliland village was broken only by kerosene lanterns, and the occasional headlights of a car jouncing over bumpy dirt roads. Two Somali nurses in white lab coats, Koos and Khush, moved ahead of Annalena in the shadows between wards.

The phlegmy cough of tuberculosis sounded louder at night, when there were fewer village sounds to mask the noise of disease. During the day, cacophony reigned. Children chanted the Koran, patients called for assistance, nurses debated the merits of certain medications, and cooks shouted for more rice or boiling water. The *adhan*, the Islamic call to prayer, rose above it all. But now quiet fell as residents of Borama ducked into their homes, away from mosquitoes and hyenas and the mountain chill. Now, in the hush of night, the coughs of the sick echoed across the courtyard.

Annalena stepped out of the corner ward, brisk but never impatient, at least never with the sick. There was still work to do – there was always work to do. She oversaw two hundred patients sleeping inside the hospital, the dozens packed into these huts, and five hundred outpatients, many of whom called the sixty-year-old Italian woman *hooyo*, or mother.

Annalena's auburn hair had long ago turned silver from age, stress, and trauma. Her blue eyes were the same clear-sky shade as the blue of the Somali flag. She was the sole white woman at the hospital, and the only Christian, and she bore no outward symbol of her faith. The only physical evidence of Annalena's spiritual conviction was tucked away in a secret satchel in her bedroom, controversial and dangerous, and only a few people in the world knew it was there.

It was nearly 8:30 p.m. on Sunday night. The last call to prayer, *isha*, had sounded an hour after dusk and most of the hospital employees had gone home hours ago. Amina Dahiye, the deaf school teacher who had been nearly dead the first time she met Annalena in Kenya, was home with her husband. Abdillahi, who had followed Annalena from Mogadishu, was at the market. He had been restless earlier in the day and Annalena had given him a handful of cash and sent him to buy biscuits and burn off energy. Shaatos, who would show me photos of Annalena when I visited him a decade later in the Netherlands, was home with his wife, Salwa.

The darkness made work at the hospital more difficult, but each patient's needs for the coming night had to be met. Fresh drinking water, a cool cloth on the forehead, a physical presence to remind the sick they didn't suffer alone. There was no need to rush home. Annalena wasn't tired – she had trained herself to sleep four hours a night. She wasn't hungry – she fasted so often her body no longer ached or trembled with weakness from hunger.

Years later a green sign in the street – faded, rusted, balanced atop two scrawny, crooked poles like the knobby legs of a tuberculosis patient – would designate the rectangular beige buildings with red roofs the ANNALENA TB HOSPITAL BORAMA. For now, the hospital was simply called the tuberculosis hospital and needed no sign.

People in town differed in what they thought Annalena did there. She may have been curing tuberculosis, which Somalis didn't call tuberculosis. They called it a cough. Or, she may have been infecting people with tuberculosis, spreading the curse around so she could get more personal publicity and money from Western sources. She may have been giving medicine to people with HIV or she may have been putting HIV into the water. She may have been giving children deworming medications or she may have been injecting them with unspeakable diseases. People said she was a nun, a missionary, a saint, a doctor, a spy. They wanted to define her, but Annalena could not be contained in a neat, single category.

The blue and white gate of the hospital didn't exist in 2003 either. There was a wall, but it was low, barely waist-high – low enough for a goat to jump over, low enough for a passerby to peer inside – made of roughhewn and sporadically placed stones and topped with nothing. No glass, no barbed wire, no metal spikes. Years later the stones would be replaced by cement and the wall raised several feet using handmade bricks. Barbed wire would top the wall. Pink plastic bags would occasionally snag on the wire and camels would munch on the bags.

Annalena had a wall around her house and a guard, Rashid. He sat at the gate during the day and slept just inside it with a gun under his bed like all the other guards who worked for foreigners in Borama. There were fewer than ten of these guards, fewer than ten compounds housing Westerners. The wall at Annalena's house was higher than the one at the hospital, the guard well-armed. But Annalena wasn't at home.

Aqals filled nearly all available space inside the hospital wall. These traditional Somali huts stood like cloth-covered termite mounds growing from dust. Each one housed a patient, maybe a family member or two, a small bundle of clothes and biscuits and paperwork tied up in a plastic bag, the papers thin and the words faded from being overly handled by anxious patients. The sick who slept in these huts were nomads who preferred sleeping outside to the metal beds, mattresses, and mosquito nets inside the hospital. Annalena would go home soon, maybe drink some tea, read her Bible and pray, write letters to her family and friends in Italy, sleep.

Two gunmen approached. Or was it one gunman? An AK-47 pointed at her head. Or was it a pistol? And when, exactly, during their encounter was it directed at her head? They may have spoken, and she may have recognized them, though the darkness would have made it hard to be certain. Koos and Khush walked toward a second ward of tuberculosis patients only a few yards away, but the huts blocked their view of the clearing and the nurses didn't know they should be watching Annalena. Koos was in Borama temporarily, on an internship. She had come from the Edna Adan Hospital in Hargeisa. She didn't know she would spend the next few days in jail.

Annalena Tonelli stood facing the gun alone. She knew the nurses were there, she knew the patients were there, 377 of them. She knew Dr. Qaws was there, a Somali doctor who lived nearby and worked closely with her. She knew there were guards and a few other employees lingering inside the hospital compound. But she stood alone with the gun in front of her and tuberculosis behind her, one woman caught between violence and disease. It wasn't the first time she had faced guns and it wasn't the first time Dr. Qaws would rush to help her. After thirty-four years in the Horn of Africa, Annalena had come to expect violence and little surprised her, though much grieved her.

There were no street lamps and many homes didn't have electricity. For those who had electricity, it remained on for a few hours in the morning and a few hours in the early evening. By now, most people had extinguished their charcoal cooking fires and turned down their kerosene lanterns. By sunrise, the first call to prayer of the day would waken residents of Borama with the amber morning light. "Prayer is better than sleep. Allah is great. Come to prayer." It would wake them to a changed reality.

I don't remember what I was doing, a few blocks away, while Annalena waited in the hospital compound with the muzzle of a gun pointed at her head, waiting to see which way this particular confrontation would go. Probably my three-year-old twins were sleeping beneath their respective blue and pink mosquito nets. Probably I had just burned a pot of popcorn and over-salted it and my husband and I picked out the edible kernels while we watched a movie projected onto the bare wall of our office. It was the end of a long day.

In the morning I had trekked to the market over boulders and cacti and past herds of camels and women pounding grain into flour. Meat hung in freshly butchered slabs from metal hooks and vendors halfheartedly waved stick brooms to ward off flies and cats. Onions, tomatoes, and garlic formed pyramids on top of burlap sacks spread over the ground. I passed my neighbor Habsan, who sold the service of grinding meat together with chopped onions, chili peppers, and cilantro.

At home, I had studied the Somali language in the afternoon and boiled water to give the twins a warm bath in a pink and white plastic bucket. I didn't know I should have been packing a suitcase.

My husband, Tom, taught physics at Amoud University, a twenty-minute drive from the village. Both of us were exhausted from maneuvering through this culture that remained strange and confusing even though we had already lived here eight months.

Matt Erickson also taught at Amoud, history and English. While Annalena stood in the compound, he sat at home on a red and gold couch with his wife, Martha, also watching a movie. There wasn't anything else to do. We had been told to stay inside after dark, for our safety. Annalena had presumably been told the same thing, but Annalena didn't follow these self-protectionist rules.

I didn't hear the sirens that night, probably because of the movie soundtrack. I didn't know that I, like the rest of Borama, would wake to a different reality. Matt and Martha did hear the sirens, but it was after dark. They were American, this was Somalia. Everyone had a gun except the foreigners, and we all knew better than to move toward sirens. The Ericksons didn't step outside their gate or even crack the front door, which opened in the direction of the hospital. They didn't glance down the block. They didn't connect the sirens with their neighbor Annalena or the tuberculosis hospital.

My housekeeper, Halimo, arrived on time the next morning. She removed her *niqaam*, the black veil that covered her face except for her eyes, and hung it on a nail in the kitchen. She told me that Annalena Tonelli had been struck and was being driven to Hargeisa. She said this with the utmost composure and started boiling water for dishes. My Somali was weak and the word *dil* could either mean to strike or to kill. I made assumptions about which meaning Halimo intended. Martha heard the news from Dr. Qaws and she called me. I had been wrong about my assumption.

The next ten days would shape the rest of my life, as Annalena's story collided with my own.

1

The Tuberculosis Holy Grail

IN 2003, I DIDN'T KNOW MUCH about Annalena and I knew even less about tuberculosis, the disease Annalena battled in Borama. For most of human history, TB was a death sentence. By the early 1900s, it had killed one out of every seven human beings to walk the planet. Today many people believe TB has been eradicated, but this airborne and contagious disease is deadlier and more widespread than ever.

TB is a wasting disease, called "the captain of death" by ancient Greeks. In the 1800s it was known as consumption because of how victims appeared to be consumed from within, betrayed by their own bodies. People grew thin until their cheekbones seemed to be all that was left of their faces. Their eyes bulged or sank into their sockets. Flesh "wasted off their faces and throats."[1] Their bodies shook with wracking, bloody coughs and they developed so much pain in the chest they couldn't get out of bed. Agonizingly, they drowned in their own liquified lung tissue.

When Annalena arrived in the Horn of Africa many Somalis, especially in rural areas, believed no good Somali ever had tuberculosis. Somalis coughed until their heads throbbed and their abdominal muscles ached. Night fevers made them sweat into their blankets and blood trickled from their lips onto their pillows. Whole families died from weight loss, weakness, trouble breathing. But no one died from tuberculosis. Their bodies bent and contorted as they coughed deep, chest-rattling coughs. They wiped blood from their mouths with the back of their hands. They had *qufac*, a cough. They never had *tibisho*, a Somalicized word from the Italian for tuberculosis.

TB was a punishment sent on illegitimate children, unfaithful spouses, and bad Muslims. It was a curse cast by jealous enemies, prideful relatives, or greedy neighbors. It was caused and spread by the hand of Allah either as a test of faith or as punishment for sin, the most common "sin" associated with *tibisho* was being born out of wedlock. Belief in this kind of causation doubled the suffering of Somalis who coughed and died of tuberculosis, adding spiritual guilt and the suspicion of their community to the agony of sickness.

With a simple, undiagnosed cough a person could remain in their home and community. Labeled with TB, they could no longer share the communal plate of rice or the communal cup of camel's milk. Others would not come close, afraid of the sinful and polluted air surrounding the sick person. Some believed TB was hereditary and could be passed down as far as six generations. They would then refuse marriages and reject children born to families rumored to have a sick member. To keep the curse from spreading, Somalis abandoned sick family members. Sometimes they left them beside acacia trees in the desert; sometimes they dropped them at the doors of remote, unstaffed pharmacies; sometimes they kicked them out of the house.

Eviction was, and is, especially dangerous for women. Nasra Odhwai, a TB patient near Garissa, an ethnically Somali town in Kenya's Northern Frontier District (NFD),[2] was kicked out of her home.[3] She slept outside the hut and in the middle of the night four men attacked and raped her. None of her family or neighbors came to her rescue. One of the attackers, Abdirahman Olow, later contracted TB himself and confessed to having raped at least twenty women who had been evicted. Harun Hussein, the regional TB deputy director said "almost all women brought to the health center" claimed they were attacked, beaten, and raped.

"The situation is fueled by community rejection of the TB patients," Hussein said.

The stigma, isolation, and abandonment that accompanied TB made an official medical diagnosis worse than death for Somalis. In the late 1960s, when Annalena arrived, there was no effective cure for TB among Somalis anyway. Better to cough, spread the cough, and die than to suffer the consequences of admitting to an incurable disease.

The Western world had had viable TB treatments for a quarter century, since the introduction of streptomycin in 1944. But these treatments required a hospital stay or regular doctor supervision for twelve to eighteen months. To be effective, the pills needed to be taken in a strict regimen.

Most Somalis in the Kenyan NFD were nomadic. They relished open spaces, freedom of movement, and autonomy. They refused to stay inside a building or follow doctor's orders on the timing of medications. They followed the sun, the Islamic prayer times, and the seasons, not clocks. If they had relatives who also coughed, they shared any pills they had; they couldn't imagine not sharing their resources. The pills could also have side effects ranging from nausea to hearing loss; people couldn't see the value of pills that made them vomit. Sometimes TB pills showed up for sale in the local markets. TB treatment was thus rendered ineffective among Somalis, and with pills in the market or treatment started and abandoned, there was a growing risk of drug resistance.

Even if people had been inclined to seek medical treatment, in 1969 there was only one hospital in the entire NFD – an area making up a third of Kenya's territory – and it lacked a tuberculosis ward. Patients slept two and three to a bed. Lepers and pregnant women, people with broken bones or snake bites, and people with TB shared beds, rooms, sheets, pillows, and utensils.

Instead, Somalis turned to faith, relying on traditional healers known as *maalins*. The sick came to *maalins* in droves, willing to try anything for a cure, anything other than staying inside a hospital for a year and a half. A visit to the *maalin* also spared people the curse and stigma of a tuberculosis diagnosis.

Maalins gathered the bitter leaves of the wanzilo tree, boiled the leaves with water, and the sick person inhaled the healing steam. A sheikh might write Koranic verses on a piece of paper, grind it with water drawn from the well of Zamzam in Mecca, and force the sick person to drink the water.

Specifically for curing a cough, *maalins* offered camel's milk to induce urination and defecation, to clear the stomach. People relied on special diets such as eating an entire animal ritually sacrificed, liver, eggs, *muuqmaad* (a beef jerky-like dried meat soaked in butter and buried underground for weeks or months to ferment), or boiled animal fat. The sheikh or a parent, most often the mother, might use a burning technique. She spun a stick with a rounded tip against a piece of wood until the tip smoked and would then burn the skin of the sick along the stomach, chest, cheeks, or back – wherever the fever seemed strongest.

The 1950s and 60s were the heyday of global TB research, and Kenya was the central hub in Africa. Scientists, fresh off the thrilling discovery of antibiotics, experimented with combination therapies that would cure TB without rendering patients immune to the antibiotics. But despite years of concentrated effort, Kent Pierce, director of the TB program in Kenya, "mournfully reported in 1961, that after five years of hard work, 'It cannot be claimed with any degree of confidence that the problem shows signs of diminishing.'"[4]

Somalis, in particular, were challenging to treat. Dr. W.S. Haynes, who ran the Port Reitz Tuberculosis Hospital in Mombasa, on the Kenyan coast, described Somalis as patients who refused to cooperate, refused to stay put, argued with doctors, and denied their diagnosis. They often presented themselves to the hospital at such a late stage of disease that they died soon after admittance, reinforcing the belief that Western medicine was a farce.

Haynes's fellow doctors refused to admit Somalis to Port Reitz without the recommendation of a respected physician, and he supported that decision. They couldn't waste limited medicine and staff on people who wouldn't follow through or cooperate. This meant Somalis had no place to go.

Somalis weren't seeking treatment, but neither were they staying quarantined. They remained nomadic and crossed international borders with impunity. They moved to urban centers like Nairobi and Mogadishu and Addis Ababa. They carried tuberculosis everywhere they went.

If there were truly no way to treat nomads with TB, scientists knew they were looking at an eventual global pandemic. After decades of scattered treatment and inconsistent antibiotic courses, multi-drug resistance was on the rise. Soon TB could become impossible to cure with any number of drugs, money, or interventions.

Scientists in Kenya said, "A viable system of domiciliary care in which patients reliably took their medicine and stayed out of the hospital became the holy grail of TB treatment. But such a thing did not yet exist in Kenya and because of this . . . there was a potentially massive problem in the works."[5]

The NFD, in particular, had no standard treatment practice for tuberculosis. In Garissa, it was so common for people to leave in the middle of treatment that the clinic created a "refusal of care" form. Patients only needed to fill in the blanks and sign with their thumb print that they understood the risks.

> I, Ado Jabane – Rer Afgab [of the Afgab family] was admitted to the Garissa TB Center in 1958. I agreed to undertake the full course of treatment, but now I want to return to my manyatta. I fully realize that I do this at my own risk, and it has been explained to me that the course of treatment is not complete. I still wish to return home. I fully realize that if TB returns then it will be entirely my own fault and responsibility.
>
> Read over and carefully explained to Ado Jabane
> District Commissioner, Garissa: (signature)
> In the presence of the DC and of Ado Jabane

The message was repeated in Swahili. This form is one of dozens on file at the Kenyan National Archives, one of thousands printed and signed at the Garissa TB Center.

The contributing factors to so many Somalis defaulting were the time frame, the treatment method, the side effects, and the mandatory restriction of movement.

Dr. J. Aluoch said, "Thiazine 12–18 months, supplemented by an initial month or two of streptomycin is not suitable to Somalis. They are used to rapid cures for all their ailments. Eighteen months is a big joke."[6]

Inpatient treatment seemed necessary because the nomadic nature of the Somali lifestyle made it impossible to expect people to return on a regular schedule to a clinic, or for medical staff to pursue patients. But inpatient treatment was also exactly what made Somalis stay away.

Tuberculosis is a community issue. If not treated and cured, one person, like Ado Jabane, could infect ten to fifteen people per year – or more, if they lived in close quarters or had already compromised immune systems. In *Discovering Tuberculosis*, Christian W. McMillen writes, "Everyone is at risk. Individual death is only part of the problem."[7]

That death is an agonizing one. For some, death comes quickly. An abscess on the lung bursts or an intestine erodes, or a major artery explodes. The victim drowns in his own blood. The most common form destroys the lungs and the space fills with fluid, pus, or fungal infections, leading to rales, a crackling, wet breathing. The chest fills up with blood and this fluid, causing that cough. "The lungs are . . . sloshing around in the chest. Cough that up, even in microscopic, impossible-to-see droplets, near other people and they have a very good chance of getting TB too. Eventually liquid entirely replaces the lungs and the suffering patients can't get enough oxygen, and respiratory failure occurs. It's painful, it's drawn out, it's an awful way to die."[8]

The final goal, according to Dr. Aluoch, had to be short-term chemotherapy. But formal programs, it seemed, would never work. After forty years of respiratory therapy work, one medical professional, Scott Karsten, said, "I've learned that the only thing that works is relationship."

Someone needed to find that scientific holy grail of treating nomads, or an international health crisis was at hand.

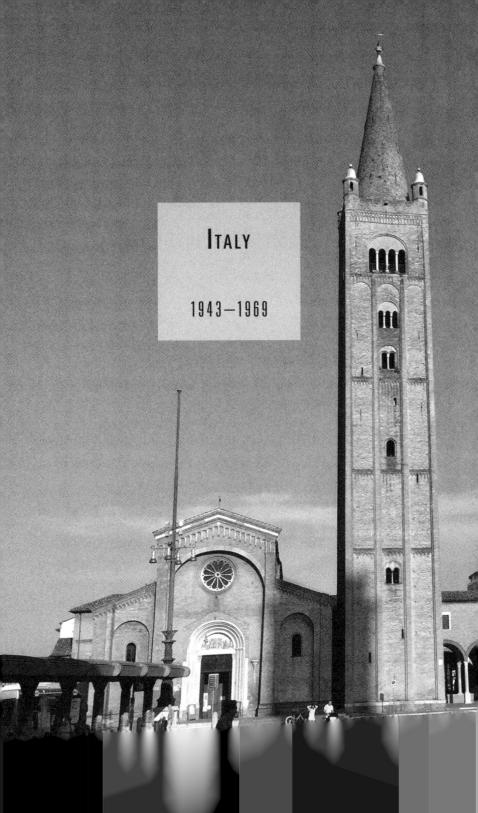

Italy

1943—1969

2

Gandhi and a Prostitute

AT FOUR O'CLOCK IN THE MORNING Annalena Tonelli biked across the town of Forlí, Italy, with schoolbooks in her backpack and a knife in her pocket. She carried the knife out of obedience, not fear – no one would ever accuse Annalena of being afraid. Her father, Guido, was afraid for her and the only way she could leave home alone in the dark at such a dangerous hour was if she carried that knife. Since he placed this single condition on her, Annalena complied. She biked across the cobblestone streets to her friend's house, where they studied for upcoming high school exams.

The streets weren't actually very dangerous, but Guido and Teresa Tonelli had lived through World War II. In 1944, Fascists denounced partisans in the Emilia-Romagna region. The partisans were captured and executed by the Nazis. A corpse swung from each lamppost that circled the central square, Piazza Aurelio Saffi, near where Annalena now biked.

Jews and sympathizers, the exact number unknown, had their hands tied behind their backs and were shot at the Forlí Airport. At the time of the airport killings, Annalena was six months old. She would nearly lose her own life during another airport massacre, forty years later and a world away.

Guido trusted Annalena to be safe and she had an excellent academic record to maintain, so he allowed her to go out. But images like bodies hanging from lampposts and corpses at the airport are hard to shake, and so he insisted on the knife. The time, hours before sunrise, wasn't early for Annalena. She read that humans spend, on average, a third of their life asleep: twenty-five years total. She determined not to waste her time sleeping and began training her body. It was stubborn and wanted to sleep; she fought back. She called her body "Brother Donkey," as Francis of Assisi had called his, and refused to give in.

Morning fog blurred the outlines of buildings and trees, muting lights and casting mysterious shadows over familiar neighborhoods as Annalena biked. "I must be crazy for how I love fog," she later wrote to her brother Bruno, from Kenya. "It is probably the usual enthusiasm for all the things God created."[1]

It wasn't just the fog that she loved about her bike rides, it was the solitude. "I remember walking and biking alone," she wrote. "Silence broken only by the flight of birds, singing cicadas, bumblebees. Once I came to a remote cemetery. How many times did I dream of being buried in a remote, isolated place?"[2]

An Italian proverb says, "Cesena to sing, Forlí to dance." Annalena, a good Forlívesi, loved to dance. She loved the cha-cha-cha and when the twist came to Italy, she was among the first of her peers to adopt it. But she wouldn't dance with boys. "Never for boys," Bruno said. "She never dressed up or performed for them. Just for fun with her friends."

When Annalena was seventeen, the family spent a month at the Adriatic Sea. School friends came to see her. As soon as she saw them approaching, she rushed into the water. They called to her, but she ignored them and stayed in the water for hours, until they were tired and bored and returned home. Once they left, she emerged from the water. She couldn't understand the draw she had on people and was, according to Bruno, totally blind to her beauty.

"I can't understand why, when I speak, I seem to be like a snake charmer," she told him. "I don't know why they look at me like this."

To Bruno, it was obvious: she was charismatic, fun-loving, full of ideas, and ready for adventure. She was beautiful, feminine, and dignified. David Brown, who would visit her in Somalia, called her aristocratic. And, she was intelligent. The Tonellis joked that in 1943, the year she was born, the hospital gave out a lot of extra brains to the babies. She also commanded obedience, or at least acquiescence. It could be easier to go along with her than to argue.

Her sisters knew this well. She and her two sisters shared a bedroom and their two brothers shared a room. The girls, Viviana, Mila, and Annalena, had small tables separating their beds. Annalena kept a lamp on her table and read late into the night.

"Turn off that annoying light," one of the sisters would say. "We can't sleep."

Annalena refused. She wanted to read, so she would read. Eventually her sisters learned to fall asleep with the light on, yielding to Annalena's "iron will," as her nephew Andrea Saletti put it.

Annalena was born too late to fully appreciate the horror of World War II, but the town of Forlí had stories.

The battle that finally freed Forlí from Nazi and Fascist control left Forlí ravaged. The Nazis blew up all the prominent towers. First the Civic Tower crashed down into the Teatro Communale. Ten minutes later the clock tower exploded. Ten minutes after that, the sound of a bell ringing seemed to call people to worship while it plummeted forty-two feet through the cathedral, shattering wooden beams on the way down.

By the time Annalena studied for her high school exams, the churches were restored and the bodies mostly forgotten. The people of Forlí had regained the character they were known for across Italy: that they had fire at the roots of their temperament.

Still, some memories remained, especially in an area known as Casermone. During the war the cathedral had housed over three hundred refugees. When it was destroyed, the people fled to Casermone, an intricate weave of narrow streets and rundown housing that was home to prostitutes, people with disabilities, abandoned children, thieves, and bullies. Probably many of them were sick, their lungs slowly turning to liquid while they coughed themselves to death. Until the end of high school, Annalena didn't know Casermone existed.

"No one knew," Maria Teresa told me. I had assumed Annalena grew up in a family focused on helping the poor or that she volunteered through the local parish and that this was how she found Casermone. But according to Maria Teresa, the church wasn't helping the people there, schools weren't helping, the government did almost nothing, and Annalena's family would have preferred she stay away.

"Who formed her?" Maria Teresa said, anticipating my question. "Where did she learn?"

Maria Teresa, Annalena's closest friend, sat next to me, our knees almost touching under a metal desk. She wore a modest, navy-blue polyester dress with buttons up the front.

The material between buttons bulged and stretched over her round belly. Her eyes were animated and sharp, bright enough to shine through her oversized, tinted glasses. She would wear this dress every time I saw her. She pronounced my name with a strong Italian accent, "Raqueley," and she usually shouted it. I liked her immediately. I had asked if Annalena was raised in a strong church community.

"The church had too many boundaries and limits," Maria Teresa said.

"She was too strong for the church," Bruno said. He sat next to his wife, Enza, across the desk from Maria Teresa and me. We were in the offices of the Comitato, an organization Annalena founded during her university years to fight world hunger.

"She was in love with people and with Jesus Christ, but not through the traditional church," Bruno said.

"She didn't follow a normal Catholic path," Maria Teresa said. "She met poor people and it was a call from them."

If she wasn't following a path laid out by her local community or family and she wasn't working within the bounds of the church, what or who launched Annalena into what would become thirty-four years of radical commitment to the poorest of the poor?

The answer came immediately to Maria Teresa's lips. "Gandhi, Gandhi, Gandhi."

Annalena met Gandhi in books during high school and took his writings so seriously she eventually referred to him as her "second gospel."

Maria Teresa said, "She learned from Gandhi that to love one must willingly and deliberately strip away self and restrict one's own needs."

Maria Teresa emphasized how scandalous this admiration of Gandhi was – that if Annalena had lived hundreds of years ago she would have been either excommunicated or burned at the stake for such a heresy. But Maria Teresa went on to loosely quote several of Annalena's favorite sayings of Gandhi's, sayings that she, too, had been radically changed by. "True religion is reflected in love for and service to man." "Our true teacher is every suffering man or woman. No act of worship is more pleasing to God than serving the poor." And the words that profoundly impacted both Annalena and Maria Teresa: "You have to be ashamed of rest and a hearty meal when on earth there is a single man or woman without work and without food. It is to eat stolen food."

According to Bruno, from the time Annalena started reading Gandhi, she stopped doing the twist. She stopped listening to music. She didn't take an extra glass of water and would rarely sit down to a full meal. "She never wanted to take more than the poor would have," Bruno said. This was around the same time that Annalena began training her body, her Brother Donkey, to sleep four hours a night.

And it was the years of the Second Vatican Council, the early 1960s. Roberto Gimelli, a friend of Annalena's from her years at the University of Bologna, said, "Annalena is incomprehensible if not properly placed in her time."

Her time was a decade of radical shifts in Catholic attitudes toward lay people and global issues. For the first time in over four hundred years, church theology was seriously reexamined and updated. One of the most obvious changes was that the church no longer required Mass to be conducted in Latin. Dialogue with other religions was encouraged and antipathy toward Protestants faded into respect. Also, lay people were encouraged to live out missional, apostolic vocations both locally and globally.

"All who work in or give help to foreign nations must remember that relations among people should be a genuine fraternal exchange in which each party is at the same time a giver and a receiver," declared Pope Paul VI in *Apostolicam actuositatem*.³ "Travelers, whether their intent is international affairs, business, or leisure, should remember that they are itinerant heralds of Christ wherever they go, and act accordingly." In short, believers wouldn't have to become nuns or priests to serve the poor or play a meaningful role in the spiritual life of their communities.

As a non-Catholic, I asked Giorgio Bertini, the Catholic bishop of Djibouti and another friend of Annalena's, to explain the impact this had on the church of Annalena's generation.

"Catholics were always committed to the poor," Bishop Giorgio said, "but more at an official level. People were interested in liturgy, catechism. But the Second Vatican Council opened things up and made Catholics rediscover what was practiced by our best saints. What should be part of daily Christian life, not relegated to a religious order."

"We are called to serve," he said. "Lay people, too. And not passively but actively. The Council," he paraphrased Pope John XXIII, "opened windows so fresh air could come into the church."

Annalena's Catholic service began with FUCI, the Italian Catholic Federation of University Students, at the University of Bologna. Roberto Gimelli, a nuclear engineering student and fellow member of FUCI, said he knew right away that Annalena was different.

I sat with him, again in the Comitato offices. Roberto was mostly bald, with wispy white hair and gentle brown eyes. His voice was thick, as though syrup coated his throat.

"We studied the new types of engagement of young lay people," he said. "But our study was a serious, academic study – until the arrival of Annalena. She made a detour and it was a moment of rupture and division, a different way of thinking for FUCI. With Annalena, we began to work with, and live near, the poor. This was shocking. But every one of us recognized that Annalena was an example of the gospel, of Christianity."

Annalena started collecting old rags and newspapers. She loaded them into the basket on her bicycle to cart around Forlí to recycle or resell. She bombarded (Roberto's word) churches with a film called *Mary and the Ants*, about world hunger, which eventually led to the foundation of the Comitato.

Maria Teresa said Annalena would, with a faint smile on her lips, suggest the most difficult and uncomfortable situations, like the time she proposed FUCI students spend a day at the Istituto Santa Teresa di Ravenna, for the mentally ill and disabled. She introduced a motto from Don Lorenzo Milani, "I care," which was a stark contrast to the Fascist motto *me ne frego*, "I don't give a damn." Caring and sharing is what Annalena expected students and her own siblings to do, when they followed her around Forlí.

But the most radical thing Annalena did, and the activity that most directed her future life choices, began with a chance encounter with a prostitute. Other than a brief mention of meeting this woman outside a shanty town, it isn't clear how Annalena got involved at Casermone. But what is clear to Bruno, Maria Teresa, and Roberto is how shocked they were at her regular forays into this dark and dangerous slum.

Dilapidated buildings – once a monastery, then a military barracks, then a refuge for war victims and dysfunctional families – Casermone consisted of long, dank corridors, garbage-strewn yards, and the echo of hostile voices. Residents generally hated affluent people like Annalena, so Roberto, then president of FUCI, decided anyone visiting had to go in pairs and there had to be one male. Annalena went alone, after dark. Roberto couldn't stop her.

Annalena took children from Casermone to medical appointments; she paid school fees; she even clipped toenails. The phone at her house would ring, someone would demand wood or coal, and off Annalena rushed.

Maria Teresa worked with children, teaching them in the afternoons, to help Annalena bear the burden of caring for the people in Casermone. Annalena's parents weren't happy about all the time she spent there, instead of on her studies.

"People would say these poor people have no mind, no heart, nothing," Maria Teresa said. "But there we found the sobering truth. The people who have no one to care for them, they become thieves and troubled. But others, who have someone to care for them, can flourish." She paused. "To flourish. To make others flourish, that was our ideal."

Annalena and Maria Teresa entertained the idea of moving into Casermone, but Annalena had brought the slum to the attention of city officials by inviting a newspaper photographer. His published photos shamed the city into closing the housing complex. Families were moved to safer, more stable houses, but the move had the unfortunate effect of dispersing what had been a tight-knit community. Since the two women could no longer move there, Maria Teresa said, "We started to think about a place where we could live poor, literally, among the people. Not to assist them but to share with them – the poverty, the risks of life, the diseases."

Maria Teresa's contrast between assisting and sharing struck me. Though my own family had moved to the Horn of Africa, I never dreamed of living like the poor. I didn't even dream of living among them. No thank you. I had a dream of helping them, swooping in to teach a skill or to bring some equipment. Actual identification with the poor, taking on the risks and dangers and stresses of their lives, held little appeal. Surely service was enough.

Such attitudes turn identification with the poor and helping them into a dichotomy, rather than two aspects of the same thing, which Annalena would come to define as love. I thought that to help effectively, I needed to remain slightly outside, slightly above, so I could retain my own health, my connections to donor organizations, my physical safety. This was a simple justification to make, and it was easier and infinitely more comfortable.

But Maria Teresa demonstrated the transformational way in which living among the poor *was* assisting them simply by bearing one another's burdens, offering dignity, building authentic relationships. The poor would become friends, not projects; community, not numbers to evaluate. They would cease to be "the poor" and became individuals with names and unique stories and personalities.

Annalena decided she couldn't give herself completely to her ideal of sharing with the poor if she stayed in Italy.

Her family pressured her to use the law degree she had studied for, but the more Annalena learned about life as a lawyer, the less appealing it seemed. She preferred to drop out of school and move, probably to India.

One day Annalena said to her mother, Teresa, "I am no longer interested in my degree. I will never be a lawyer. It would mean entering a life I would never enjoy."

"You finish," her mother said. "Then you go anywhere. You want to go to India? Go. You want to go to Africa? Go. But first, you graduate."

Annalena obeyed her parents and completed her law degree, with an emphasis on juvenile delinquency. During this time, she met Pina Ziani, a woman twenty years her senior who had spent four years in Somalia serving lepers. Annalena saw in Pina the incarnation of her desire to serve the poor. She even called Pina her "second soul." Roberto said Annalena followed Pina around like a puppy.

When Pina learned of Annalena's desire to live abroad, she suggested Annalena go to Kenya and secured a teaching contract for her at the Chinga Girls Secondary School in Nyeri, central Kenya, a position with the Consolata Mission.

"My family didn't want this," Annalena later told a journalist, "so of course I took the first chance."[4]

In the days before Annalena departed for Kenya, she and Maria Teresa perched at the top of a short, cobbled street that sloped sharply down toward the sea. Annalena recalled their conversation in a letter from the barren desert of Wajir, Kenya:

> A majestic calm deep blue night sky with a few stars. The two of us were kidnapped by beauty and you were telling me about a cascade of other beauties around the world. Mountains, valleys, woods, oceans green as emeralds, ancient lands. We were breathless, as if we did not belong to this world. You asked how I could do without all of this, to deprive myself. And I was desperately trying to make you understand that it was not as you said, and that yes, I could live to the end of my days without any green thing. It is the power of imagination, Maria Teresa. . . . I hear these words over and over and summon images of the sea.[5]

Memories were all Annalena would have of the sea for the next seventeen years.

A bronze bust of Annalena hung on the wall over Maria Teresa's head at the Comitato and I glanced at it while we talked. I snapped a photo of it and Maria Teresa waved dismissively.

"This is so ugly," she said. "But someone sent it to us, so we hung it up."

The bust depicted an image of what I started to call "Saint Annalena," one of the most widely circulated photographs of her. In it, she wears a blue scarf with a thin, lighter blue hem the same shade as her eyes, draped over graying hair. Age spots mark her temples. She smiles without showing her teeth. The fine lines of her cheekbones and nose have softened, wrinkles spider out from the corners of her eyes. She gazes into the distance and I imagine she is thinking of Wajir, her "paradise on earth." A light hits the side of her head and casts a glow over her hair and face. She looks like an elderly, Italian Virgin Mary. It is a pose. The serene smile, the steady gaze, the halo, crafted to present an image of a woman people would attempt to beatify. Crafted to mask the fury, stubborn nature, and earthiness of a woman few understood. And yet, it also conveys a sense of faith and confidence, equally true of Annalena. This was the Annalena I thought I was researching, the holy and superhuman.

"I hate this picture that makes her look like a saint," one of her coworkers later told me. "If you have a photo of Annalena, you need one of her laughing."

"She was not a saint," Maria Teresa said, that first day we talked in the Comitato. "As long as we are alive, we won't let the church take her."

She couldn't be a doctor, according to her brother Bruno; that was a job for him. She couldn't be a missionary, also according to Bruno; she was too strong for the church. She couldn't be a nun; later she would write that she wanted to be married to the desert and to desert people, specifically Somali nomads. People would call her a doctor, a missionary, and a nun. And, they would call her a saint. Were Maria Teresa, Bruno, and Enza wrong? Should Annalena be made into a saint?

That was how I thought of her, at first. I only knew the high points in Annalena's life. I knew nothing of the dark valleys, her secret and controversial compromises.

I knew she had accomplished something remarkable, something about tuberculosis but also about love and faith. She lived a life I had also attempted in Somalia, but I had a growing suspicion that I had missed something essential. I couldn't yet identify it, though I knew it had something to do with what motivated Annalena, what sustained her, and how she defined success and failure.

KENYA

1969—1985

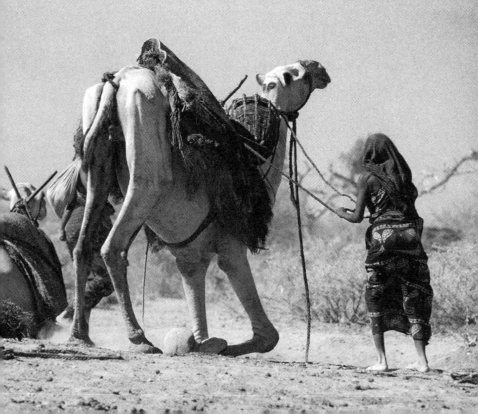

3

Desert Paradise

RELENTLESS WIND WHIPPED the desert into tornadoes of dust that curled through every crevice in the Land Cruiser carrying Annalena away from her first home in Kenya. Chinga, nestled among the green hills of Nyeri, had been beautiful, serene, and too comfortable. Annalena was moving toward need.

By the time the Land Cruiser bounced over the 250 miles and crossed the only functional bridge over the Tana River, the lush forests, mountains, and jacaranda petals of a more moderate climate were only a memory.

The dirt was no longer red, but beige and light, more like baby powder than soil. It coated Annalena's clothes and skin, settled on her eyelashes, clogged her throat, and obscured her vision. The trees were shorter here in the Northern Frontier District. Acacias, squat and leafless with flattened tops, offered scant shade and scores of three-inch-long, needle-sharp thorns. These were the thorns used by Somali midwives to sew up circumcised girls.

Human-sized termite mounds, endless rocks, and the occasional delicate plant with pale blue flowers flashed past. Somali women plucked the flowers, let them dry, then rubbed them to release small black seeds known as *haba sodah*, black cumin. They mashed the seeds with hot oil and massaged it over the bodies of people plagued by bloody, uncontrollable coughing, in hopes that the induced sweat would force out the disease, or the demons that caused it.

The Land Cruiser passed frankincense trees from which nomads gathered sap to combine with water, camel dung, and a bleaching agent from local roots to wash clothes. Village women burned the frankincense sap over charcoal to perfume their homes and attract their husbands. Annalena didn't know yet that the scent of frankincense would come to signify home. She did know that this was where she wanted to live.

Until recently, white foreigners other than British colonial officers weren't allowed to make a home in northern Kenya. Missionaries had been forbidden under colonial law because the British were afraid to do anything that might upset the precarious balance between peoples, specifically between Somali clans. In crossing the Tana River to fulfill her teaching contract in the NFD instead of at the Chinga Girls Secondary School in Nyeri, Annalena would be one of only a handful of foreigners in the north. She needed special permission from the Ministry of Education.

This wasn't difficult to obtain. No one wanted to go north.

Chinga and Nyeri were what foreigners imagined when they thought of Kenya. Tourist country. Rich, lush soil ideal for growing coffee and tea; towering trees; monkeys, giraffes, and zebras in the Kenyan National Forest; red dirt pathways that cut up steep hills. Paradise. The tea plantation countryside of Karen Blixen's 1937 memoir *Out of Africa* was exactly the kind of place Annalena had feared Kenya would be. Now she had a chance to escape.

Wajir, in the north, was historically a punishment assignment. Colonial administrators sent underlings there when they were displeased with them. Kenyans paid bribes to avoid being placed as teachers, government officials, or medical staff in Wajir.

Life in the north was harsh, and a primary source of suffering was the well water. There were high levels of mica, gypsum, amoebas, and bacteria in the water, and people came down with typhoid regularly. The health department found that the water was full of camel urine from centuries of herds gathered around Wajir's wells. A UNICEF survey declared the water in Wajir unfit for human consumption.

Undissolved crystals of mica and gypsum irritated the urinary tract, bladder, and kidneys and caused a sensation of "peeing razor blades."[1] Residents referred to a glass of Wajir water as a "cup of tears."[2]

To avoid drinking the water, people gathered rain in barrels. But even rainwater had to be consumed cautiously, as the storage tanks often held carcasses of geckos, roaches, or other drowned creatures.

A year before Annalena moved to Kenya, 3,520 cattle had been raided in the area around Wajir, and there had been a series of armed confrontations between the Degodia and the Ajuran Somali clans as they fought over grazing rights and access to wells. Lions attacked isolated nomads and snakebites were common. Temperatures soared to 105 degrees Fahrenheit and there was no electricity: no air conditioners, no fans, no way to make ice. Rain, on the rare occasions when it did fall – as little as five inches annually – could lead to catastrophic flooding.

In the NFD, an area nearly fifty thousand square miles with a population of six hundred and eighty thousand, giving birth was one of the most dangerous things a woman could do. Nomadic women labored under acacia trees in the desert, hoping to catch up with the family as soon as the baby was born. If a woman needed to be transported to a hospital, she would be loaded onto a camel and led one or two hundred miles, the baby and mother often dead upon arrival.

Tuberculosis, malaria, typhoid, cholera, and dengue fever raged. Even in places where a bit of medical intervention was possible, it was mostly ineffective due to culture, superstitions, and the limitations of people able to think only about surviving one more day, with little vision of a long-term future.

Life here was short and brutal.

The sun beat down, baking the rocky earth. There were no mountains and no bodies of water other than the murky brown river filled with catfish and crocodiles. Thirst and the hunt for shade dominated life north of the Tana River.

The region held a desolate kind of beauty, but it was a desperate beauty that bespoke the dogged human struggle to survive. Here Mother Nature and human nature seemed locked in a perpetual battle.

The expansive desert spoke to Annalena of the vastness of God. The view that stretched for miles, unhindered, made her aware of her own smallness and provided space for her eyes and imagination to roam.

Though Annalena was eager to move to Wajir, away from the ease of Nyeri, Somali residents weren't keen to welcome her. They tended to be suspicious of outsiders, especially Christian outsiders, and for good reason. They had only recently gotten rid of the British, at independence in 1960. But they had been trying to rid the Horn of Africa of infidels for over half a century.

In 1895 Muhammad Abdullah Hassan returned from Saudi Arabia to his native Somalia.

Muhammed landed in the port town Berbera and strolled through customs. A British colonial officer demanded customs tax. Muhammed asked why he should pay a foreigner for the right to enter his own country. Other Somalis at the port told the officer to ignore him, he was just a "crazy mullah." The name stuck, and Muhammed became known as the Mad Mullah.

As the Mad Mullah walked through Somaliland, he found a boarding school, established by French Catholics. Here, Somali children learned reading, writing, and mathematics – and about the Catholic faith.

The Mad Mullah asked the most basic Somali questions of the children: who their parents were and what their clan was. Somalis value lineage highly and most can recite their ancestral heritage as far as twenty generations back. One boy said his name was "John Abdullahi." The others answered that they belonged to *Reer Fader*, or the "clan of the Catholic fathers."

Muhammed was furious and tore the cross from the boy's neck.

Convinced that Christians were a threat to Somali children, culture, and religion, Muhammed turned toward a pan-Somali ideal. He would drive the Christians and colonizers into the sea and unify the Somali people with political and religious independence under Somali rule. It was a promise he failed to keep.

In a letter that echoed down through decades and found itself on pamphlets in Mogadishu during the American intervention in 1993, as well as on the lips of post-9/11 jihadists, the Mad Mullah wrote, "I have no forts, no houses, no country, I have no cultivated fields, no silver or gold for you to take – all you can get from me is war. If you wish peace, go away from my country to your own. If you wish war, stay where you are."[3]

Ultimately, Muhammed's campaign to rid Somalia of foreign infidels ended in defeat. But the sentiment that Somalia was for Somalis lived on. White, foreign non-Muslims were not welcome, or were welcomed only with great suspicion.

As Annalena neared Wajir, a hollow sound echoed across the sand. Wooden, handcrafted camel bells, unique to each camel, clacked and clattered. This sharp tap would become the background noise of Annalena's life, day and night. Camels moaned, roared, and harrumphed as they waited their turn at Qorohey, "the sunny place," where nomads watered their herds outside Wajir.

Shepherds worked in teams and sang love songs about women and camels, war and heroism.

They passed buckets made of goat or camel hide, sometimes giraffe hide, from hand to hand and poured the water into troughs. While they worked, women drew water for household needs, balancing jugs on their heads, hips, or shoulders. Sand grouse, Marabou storks, and pigeons flocked to the puddles of spilled water – so many birds that the air filled with the sound of beating wings.

Herders identified their own camel by its bell and its footprints – the size and shape of the toes and its pace. Simply by looking at the prints left in the desert sand, they knew if a camel was loaded or empty, watered or thirsty, tired, wounded, or blind in one eye. Camel owners considered themselves kings; there was no greater possession among Somalis.

Herders survived for days at a time on camel milk, which could be consumed fresh or sour without any special pasteurization, stored in containers sterilized with charcoal smoke.

Behind the scrum of camels and shepherds, Annalena could see Wajir's main mosque over the pale green palm fronds, the nomads' *aqals*, and the remnants of the Wajir Fort. The mosque bore the telltale splotches and chipped paint of a job hastily done with cheap materials, many years ago. Wind, sun, and brutal dust storms sanded the corners of buildings into rounded edges. She was home.

Maria Teresa joined Annalena on March 14, 1970. They planned to live off Annalena's teaching salary and Maria Teresa would work with disabled children. But first they needed to learn how to live in Wajir.

"Maria Teresa has the soul of a pioneer," Annalena wrote. "I have the temperament of a nomad. Everywhere feels like I am home. Wonderful!"[4]

"I was more balanced," Maria Teresa said to me, "I was Sancho Panza, with good sense. She was Don Quixote. I slept, she never slept. I wanted to eat a lot of rice, she didn't eat. I ate to fill my stomach. Not Annalena. She ate lettuce, some cheese, a few eggs, a chapatti."

On her first day in Wajir, Maria Teresa moved the gas cylinder to attach it to the stove to heat water. An insect flew up at her face.

Later that same morning, in the corner of the courtyard, she saw a snake curled up in a tight coil. A small boy holding a stick stood nearby and she called him over. He picked up a stone and with the stick and stone, like David facing Goliath, he killed the snake.

"We had everything," Maria Teresa said. "Water, lanterns, snakes."

They didn't have air conditioning and temperatures remained over 95 degrees, even at eleven o'clock at night. When I asked about a fan, Maria Teresa laughed. "Oh no. You are saying a thing that is impossible."

The house had several rooms, but the women only used one. Annalena wanted to be poor. "You cannot love the poor," she said, "without wanting to be like them."[5] She believed claiming to love the poor while remaining rich would have been welfare, not love.

"Poor, poor, poor," Maria Teresa said, about this ideal, and laughed.

The house was nearly empty of furnishings. They had two beds but, in the beginning, slept only on mats on the floor. After one night fighting off tarantulas, Maria Teresa moved her mattress onto the bed frame.

"But Annalena, she was a friend to everything," Maria Teresa said. "I jumped up onto a bed and never left it." Annalena stayed on the floor. Or sometimes, she spread her mat on top of her desk. A cushion would have been too luxurious.

"Maria Teresa," Annalena said, "if the poor don't have a bed, why should I?"

In the mornings, they woke to mountains of bugs on the ground and swept them out, to make room for more.

"The life was quite a shock at first," Maria Teresa said.

They discovered, to Annalena's dismay, that they couldn't adapt to all aspects of the life of the poor. Without a wooden door, hyenas, thieves, or lions could enter the house. Drinking only camel's milk would have left them too weak for work. They compromised with occasional bits of camel or goat meat. And though the house was simple, they kept it spotless.

"Our house was cleaner than the Wajir Hotel," Maria Teresa said proudly. "We couldn't live exactly like the poor, but we could live like the rich poor."

Their few luxuries came in the mail. Pina Ziani sent coffee, chocolate, and books. Annalena said opening the packages was like Christmas Eve. Knorr broth envelopes for soup, homegrown spices to make the beans and chewy camel meat edible, music cassettes, interesting articles, perfume samples. Annalena treasured the reading materials above everything

else and piled them on her desk, beside her students' papers
waiting to be graded.

Maria Teresa tried to be the first to peer into Pina's packages. She knew Annalena would give away everything except
the books, so she pulled out the small soaps from hotels and
the perfumes.

"I hid it all in a suitcase under the bed or behind an
armchair," she said. When she was overcome with heat and
sweat, a bit of perfume was "like a resurrection."

Annalena tried writing letters at night by lantern or moon-
light outside, but mosquitoes, scorpions, and spiders forced
her to return to the comfort of mosquito netting. Inside, her
arms stuck with sweat to the pages. "I am the inferior one
here," she wrote. "Brutalized by this climate. A sun that burns
to the edges of nausea and breaks the legs as if one had to
carry stones for hours and hours."[6] She had one word for how
she felt, crushed by the heat and the bugs and her inability to
live exactly like the poor: "Defeated."

Annalena never owned more than two or three outfits at a
time and chose simple colors, shades of blue and purple. She
wore modest, long dresses, but never covered her head, not
even in Somalia, until ordered to by elders, decades later.
Dressing modestly was more practical than philosophical. If
she didn't cover her legs, she said, she would feel embarrassed,
or naked. "We wore the Somali dress," Maria Teresa said. "The
long one. No socks, no gloves, no scarf, no slip. It was too hot."

Aqals lined the streets and the area outside Wajir, near the
wells. Annalena wandered among the huts, observing and
learning. Women constructed these temporary houses using
the pliable roots of dhumay or galool trees, a type of acacia.

Once they formed a solid structure of eight to twelve curved supports, they covered it with thinner branches. On top of those, they used torn strips of clothing to tie down mats made of tightly woven dried grasses. When families moved on, the women dismantled the houses and loaded them onto their camels, every item reusable. Rebuilding it would take half a day at the next stop.

People owned only what they could carry or load onto camels. They ate what their animals provided or what they could trade for in villages. By Western standards, Somali nomads in the NFD were chronically malnourished, uneducated, and among the poorest people in the world. But the nomads didn't view their lives through Western standards. They were rulers of the earth, fiercely attached to the land, their camels, and their people.

But, strong as nomads were, a silent scourge ravaged them and rendered them weak, unable to walk alongside their camels or build a hut. They would start to cough and lose weight; their chests burned and they lost their appetite. Whole families living in a single, cramped space woke up with blood on their lips. They were rulers of their desert domain, but they were dying.

Staff of the few humanitarian organizations operating in the NFD didn't see the blood or hear the coughs. They saw skinny people who didn't send their children to school. They saw dry ground and no agriculture. They interpreted the lack of possessions as poverty and their solutions fit into this narrative. More schools, more boreholes for wells, innovative farming methods, food donations – the elements that have comprised the core of aid for decades.

Many boreholes started as aid and development projects were never finished. The imported farming methods drew families into towns to settle, but they brought their animals and the towns were unable to support the increased grazing demands. Areas as large as six miles surrounding villages that had once been green and healthy turned to fine dust, land in which nothing would grow. Food donations meant local shopkeepers didn't earn enough from their stores. When nomads shunned educational opportunities, they were accused of ignorance, which placed the blame on them rather than on the educational system – a curriculum based on an urban and agricultural life that made no sense to nomads.

Donations came out of wealthy people's surplus: extra books, unwanted clothing, and leftover food. Rarely was much actual sacrifice required on the part of humanitarian workers, whose inconvenience was compensated with higher "hardship" posting salaries. And the aid they brought consistently failed to meet the real, felt needs of the people.

Annalena believed the problem was with selfish missionaries and secular aid workers who didn't know how to serve or how to love, who refused to be purified from their addiction to comforts and distractions, such as television and extra shoes. She wrote that if everyone loved and served well, all the orphans, the crippled, the abandoned, and the unhappy in the entire world could be gathered up and cared for.

But she herself struggled to know how to meet needs. Outside, people went hungry and thirsty and suffered from broken limbs and diseases. Inside the house, she and Maria Teresa had nutritious food. Thanks to a water pump, they had a faucet and showers; thanks to her teaching contract, economic security. Outside, people sat for hours in the shade without moving, without talking. Annalena speculated that some even stayed in their positions through the night.

Day after day Annalena and Maria Teresa gave them what they could.

"But we give them what does not cost us anything, what we would not use, the food we do not eat, the clothes we do not wear," Annalena said.[7] It was no sacrifice. The last thing Annalena wanted was what she called a castle, a place from which she could dispense education, medicine, religion. That was how she viewed secular humanitarian and missionary life – people protecting themselves, building comfortable citadels and claiming positions of power and authority.

"Our giving is so limited," Annalena said, "so choked that one cannot help but ask if it was worth it to leave our country? To transplant oneself here only to not fully give oneself away? To demand comfort and space to rest, to participate in small, discrete activities, always a little below average, always giving with a little energy or money in reserve." If that was why people came to Africa, "it would have been better to stay at home. We must do everything to give everything, to love all, serve all."[8]

I saw myself right in the middle of that paragraph. Demanding comfort, rest, always keeping a little energy and money in reserve. Would it have been better for me to stay in the United States? Is there any shame in maintaining a level of comfort, in giving just the average amount?

I wanted so much for the Annalena I read about to like me, to affirm my choices. But I had the uncomfortable sense that I would be one of the people she wrote home about, living in my big cement house inside a wall topped with broken glass, guarded by an armed young man. I was in Somalia, my husband taught at Amoud University, the only functioning higher education institution in the country at the time. We dreamed about impacting Somalia from the ground up by investing in the next generation of leaders, educators, and thinkers.

I wanted to see evidence that the choice we had made mattered, that the things we had given up would be repaid in some tangible way. The reward I wanted might look like acceptance into the community, students educated and moving into positions of leadership, meaningful relationships with locals.

It would take me years, and Annalena, to understand a better way to measure impact and success.

4

Thirst

HINTS OF A COMING DROUGHT appeared in the NFD. Droughts were so common and devastating that Somalis named them according to their characteristics. Instead of remembering the dates of birthdays or anniversaries, people said, "I was born in the second year of Haraamacune." Or, "My parents got married at the end of Siigacase." Haraamacune, the drought of 1911–12, Eater of the Forbidden Food, because to survive some people resorted to eating *haram*, Islamically unclean, food. Siigacase, the drought of 1950–1951, Blower of Red Dust, after frequent sandstorms. The drought that was coming would be called Dabadheer, Long-Tailed One, because of its longevity.

Wajir's low annual rainfall, extreme temperatures, constantly blowing dust, and distance from any significant body of water gave the town's wells an aura of the miraculous. The earth's surface was parched, the ground dry and cracked, but underneath, streams of water flowed. The water came from rain in the Abyssinian mountains, over two hundred miles away in Ethiopia. It ran underground, unseen and unacknowledged, until it met the limestone rock around Wajir and seeped upward.

A colonial officer wrote that Somalis believed the Wajir water was "possessed of peculiar properties and women who are unable to bear children are in the habit of visiting it to drink the water. While the water has certainly a laxative effect on the uninitiated, the medical officer does not consider its properties to be such as to increase female fertility; Somalis, however, believe it to be true." Whether or not the well water cured infertility was irrelevant. Women needed hope. They had no access to doctors or medical treatment, so they did what they could. It isn't as though Somali women chose amoeba-ridden water over in vitro fertilization. There was one hospital in the entire NFD and the shelves of its pharmacy were often empty. Elspeth Huxley, who wrote extensively about Kenya and the NFD, suggested, "A quasi-magical explanation of puzzling objects or events is common among almost all unsophisticated peoples."[1] But it would be a mistake to write off the Somalis Annalena met in Wajir as unsophisticated. Considering their limited options, they proved quite resourceful, brave, and creative in their quest for medicine, willing to experiment with anything. The same would be true of tuberculosis.

No rain fell in Wajir in 1969. In early 1970, Annalena and Maria Teresa were near the hospital when rain started, pouring down in sheets, like buckets of water tipped over the village. Wild with joy, they joined children in the streets. Everyone laughed and screamed and splashed in the puddles. Big, blooping drops shot down, almost violently. Annalena raised her arms and spun in circles as the fresh water caressed her skin. It rained so hard that within minutes there was enough water on the ground that women dragged metal basins into the puddles and started scrubbing clothes. Children emerged from their homes with bars of soap and bathed, despite the mud.

Now that it was raining, Annalena learned a hard lesson of the frontier. There was no vegetation or drainage ditches to hold the water and the entire region turned into a morass. Rain washed out the road between Wajir and the next major town, Garissa. Trucks overturned, toilet cisterns overflowed, and mosquitoes hatched in the puddles, bringing the threat of malaria, cholera, and typhoid. And, ironically, hunger, as slowly, slowly shelves in the *dukas* emptied because supply trucks could not make it through the water and thick mud.

The diseases never came. The rain stopped. Annalena learned that one or two rains, even a deluge, weren't enough. Thirst in the desert could never be satisfied. And what she had thought were The Rains, the official rainy season, was really just a storm. The rainy season failed again.

After the initial deluge, almost no more rain fell. By August the roads dried out and supply trucks again arrived with food and medications. The few flowers that blossomed after the rain wilted. The earth turned back into cracked clay. No rain in September and the landscape became even more burnt. Dead leaves crackled into dust and thorn bushes withered.

Doves clattered on aluminum roofs and swooped down to join sand grouse on the ground, drinking from puddles by the wells, the only place to find water. Annalena woke early to watch the birds fly over her neighbors, who gathered in four long rows to pray the morning Islamic *salat*. She watched the people bow and kneel and rise. As the sun rose, it burned so intensely white against the bleached earth and white buildings she was forced to squint before turning to her own prayers and Bible reading for the day.

By late November the rains still hadn't come. People were thirsty. November this year was the fasting month of Ramadan. For one lunar cycle, Muslims didn't eat or drink anything from sunup until sundown. Water was all people or animals could think about, but thinking about it didn't bring rain. Cows and camels started to die.

Annalena kept her eyes on the sky while she planned lessons and while she taught them. Once she thought she smelled rain and ran out of her English class to sniff the air like a dog. Nothing.

She loved the sky, even that cloudless sky. When she did brave the mosquitoes and sleep outside during the hot season, with no electricity for miles to lessen the brilliance of the stars, she would stretch out her hands and imagine she could grab hold of the stars. She called them her lullaby, singing her into the light of dawn.

She wondered why nomadic families didn't move to Wajir, nearer to the water. But nomads must keep moving. They came to Wajir for water but couldn't stay and graze. There would never be enough pastureland near the town for thousands of animals. As soon as bellies and jugs were full, the camel trains moved on. In times of drought, even as they weakened, the need to move increased. Further inland to find pasture, further from the wells. They couldn't stop for women to give birth. They couldn't stop for fevers or when someone stepped on thorns that pierced through their feet or when people coughed up blood.

People in the bush constantly looked to the sky, pulsing with heat, and hoped for rain. More than a hope even – they expected rain. Endlessly and without any reason, without a cloud or a cool breeze. They asked Allah for rain and that was enough. "Tomorrow it will rain," they would say. And while they waited, expectant and prayerful, they died of thirst and starvation.

The faith of Somalis in the NFD can seem like fatalism. It can be difficult to see the faith in it. Allah said he knew the number of his people's days; they could do nothing to prolong or shorten their lives. Taking prophylaxis for malaria or treatment for tuberculosis or abandoning one's way of life because of drought was evidence of a lack of faith. Allah could bring rain if he wanted to. He could cure diseases if that was what he had written. Allah was able to provide all things, but he was also capricious and, for his own inexplicable purposes, might withhold rain and healing. Somalis didn't question his plan or his timing. To Annalena, this wasn't fatalism but the very essence of faith: utter reliance on and loyalty to Someone outside oneself, and the willingness to conform one's life to that Someone.

Annalena came to see why Islam was a religion of the desert. This demand for submission enabled people to live, suffer, and die with dignity, knowing their lack of complaint and acceptance of all things pleased Allah. Faith didn't destroy them or weaken them – quite the opposite. They knew their own strength and, as another foreigner wrote about Somalis during a drought, faith "prevented them from wasting themselves in fury and desperation."[2]

And so, ready to accept whatever came, the people watched the skies, hoped for rain, and trusted Allah.

Annalena had another lesson of the desert coming, when the real rains began: with every blessing comes a curse. Along with the rains, disease came to Wajir.

5

Infidel

IN JANUARY 1971 the first official case of cholera on the entire African continent in seventy years was diagnosed, and before long it was in the NFD. Health department officials speculated that nomads crossing the Somali and Ethiopian borders in ever-widening hunts for water and pasture brought it into Kenya. The arrival of cholera should have been a warning sign that diseases wouldn't obey border controls. It should have provided motivation for change and development. But it was easier to blame others than to take responsibility for the disastrous medical care and water situation. The result: where there had long been no cholera, between 1971 and 2011 there were over three million cases across Africa.

Symptoms of cholera are diarrhea and severe dehydration. Treatment is a simple rehydration fluid, given either orally or through an IV. Cholera spreads twice as fast as Ebola and, left untreated, can kill within hours.

Already before the crisis, hospital care had been atrocious. Now, Annalena struggled to think of words serious enough to describe the situation. "Absurd, inconceivable, unacceptable, a tragedy, inhuman and dehumanizing. . . . For the sick, it is like an infinite punishment. We can do a little but the mass suffering weighs on the heart. For people in town there is, in theory, the hospital. I only say, in theory."[1]

People with infectious diseases slept on sheets that went unchanged between patients. They lay in their own excrement for hours, or days. The floors were filthy. Cockroaches scrambled up and down the walls and into beds. The pungent smell of sweat, unwashed bodies, blood, and human waste clung to everything. At night hens and foxes wandered between rooms looking for food and water, sometimes breaking items such as thermometers, leaving glass and mercury in their wake.

Annalena said nurses and attendants walked back and forth, "casual, relaxed, as if there was nothing to do. They chatted and drank tea, while the women worked on personal sewing projects. They know very little and do as little as possible. They pass the whole day doing almost nothing."[2] When they did visit patients, there were complaints that they were rude and careless, that they gave medications to the wrong patients or didn't pay attention.

"There is no one," Annalena wrote to her family, "and I mean no one, who takes the initiative to wash a sick person or clean urine or vomit. No one listens to the suffering, no one brings them the relief of a little water, a change of position, a word of comfort."[3] Her future colleague, Elmi Mohamed, agreed with her. "Sure, there are some good nurses, but mostly they listened to the radio and walked around."

Until the early 1970s, the hospital didn't even have electricity. The Medical Officer, Mark Wood, had a generator installed, but when it broke, it took months for someone to go to Nairobi for parts. Doctors did emergency surgeries at night by flashlight or with car headlights aimed at the operating theater. There was no equipment that required electricity, such as x-ray machines.

The combination of cholera and drought left children especially vulnerable. Those who contracted cholera or became too weak from hunger to keep up with their families were abandoned, sometimes with their mothers beside them, staring blankly ahead, stone-faced with grief. Sometimes they were left alone in a hut or beneath a tree, sometimes they were carried to Wajir. Some families promised to return after finding food and water. Some did, stumbling back to Wajir months later to find out whether or not their children had survived. Others perished or simply never returned.

Twenty-five sick children were left in the hospital and Annalena took over their care, alongside her teaching responsibilities.

"We took them home," Maria Teresa said, "and they were all supposed to die."

"So many people came with terrible stories," Maria Teresa said. "Wife, children, goats dying because of hunger and thirst and they said, 'This is the will of God. I have lost everything; it is the will of God.' This was real faith. Annalena said she had never seen such faith in our European people. That faith was a big teacher for us. We couldn't show faith like that, but, in the end, they knew we were able to love."

"Is love the same as faith?" I asked Maria Teresa. In answer, she told a story.

She and Annalena were in the bush, after the cholera, and a sheikh approached.

"Why did you stay here?" he asked. Other foreigners had fled.

Annalena said, "Because our religion is equal to love. If we really love God, we must help the last, the poorest."

"Your God asks you a difficult thing," the sheikh said. "Our religion doesn't ask such a big task. Our religion is . . ." Maria Teresa struggled to find the word.

"*Fudud*," I said.

"*Fudud!*" She laughed. "You know it. Yes, easy. Our religion is easy, that's what he said. Then he said, 'We have the true religion. You have love, we have faith.'"

Annalena saw the faith of Muslims and embraced it as authentic. She called it the most extraordinary gift she received from the desert nomads.

"Unconditional abandonment, surrender to God. A surrender which is not fatalistic, a surrender which is rock solid and anchored in God. They taught me to do everything in the name of God. *Bismillah al-Rahman, al-Rahiim.*"[4]

In answering my question about faith and love, Maria Teresa essentially said that Annalena brought together the compassion she saw in Jesus, the surrender she saw in Muslims, and her own love for the poor, and the combination produced faith. Active, living faith.

Ibrahim, a three-year-old in Annalena's care who suffered from both malnutrition and spinal tuberculosis, was gravely ill. In March, policemen had found him in the desert, dying of hunger. He clung to anyone willing to hold him and pressed his head against the person's chest. Annalena took him home from the hospital; she wanted to keep him close through the nights too, so he wouldn't die alone. When she first stretched him out on a bed, he pulled her down to lay beside him and rested his head over her heart.

"Who knows how much he has suffered. Now he just wants comfort, peace, and the security of a mother's heartbeat," she said.[5]

By early May, Ibrahim showed marked improvement. If Annalena held him on her lap, he would eat. At first it took him an entire day to finish a dish of rice, milk, and sugar, but slowly he was able to hold more in his stomach without vomiting. Eventually he wanted seconds and thirds.

And then Ibrahim died. It was three o'clock in the afternoon on May 12. He had a high fever and had contracted a "withering attack" of measles. Annalena wasn't there when he died. "First I tried to pray, then I cried. Then I tried to write, read, sleep. But I could not get anything done. Once again, it is clear that I cannot hide my head in the sand and not face reality." [6]

Most of the twenty-five children survived. Now that Annalena had been introduced to the sick, she was hooked. Tuberculosis patients caught her most powerfully. They were the ones left most often on dirty sheets, dying alone, most shunned by nurses and family members. There was no tuberculosis ward at the hospital and scant medications. At least she could give them a sip of cold water. She took the words of Jesus literally and brought water from the roof of her house, where she had a storage bucket, to the hospital to replace the dirty well water. Then, she started to treat the sick. [7]

She relied on books Bruno sent from Italy, and the knowledge of local healthcare workers, though she was dismayed by their lack of compassion and expertise. Later, she would go to Europe for training in tropical medicine, but for now she only had her books.

Tuberculosis was considered an African disease not worthy of investment, in the naive assumption that somehow Western countries would be immune. But, as Dr. Onkar Sahota, chair of London's Health Committee said in 2015, "We think TB is a disease of developing countries or of days gone by, but TB is a disease of today. It certainly was a disease of yesterday and we need to make sure it isn't a disease of tomorrow." [8] In 2015, some neighborhoods in London had higher rates of TB than almost anywhere else in the world, including Rwanda, Iraq, and Guatemala.

Compared to tuberculosis in scope, cholera and Ebola look like minor blips. Ebola killed 3,338 people between March and October of 2014. During those same months, over 600,000 died of tuberculosis in Africa alone.

"The worst disease," a Somali nomad said, "is still TB."[9]

But, as Maria Teresa said, "How can you keep a nomad in the hospital?"

One young woman, her name lost to sand and history, had suffered polio and now hovered near death from tuberculosis. Annalena sat by her side in the final hours of her life. Though they couldn't communicate in any shared spoken language, Annalena said she and this woman understood one another.

The woman's legs were limp, thin as sticks, her body so emaciated it was frightening – a rice sack filled with bones. But her face was filled with expression, an awareness. According to the dictates of her clan, she wore the black veil of a married woman, dignified in its modesty. Even though she was now divorced, she still bore the pride of a woman who had been married, once chosen. She asked Annalena, with hand gestures and her eyes, to spend the coming night in the room with her.

The woman coughed incessantly. Annalena sat beside her, bearing witness. Here was one of God's sparrows – one of Annalena's favorite words for describing the sick – falling to the ground, known by her Creator and neglected by her people. Annalena grew drowsy, the heat pushing her head down toward her chest, urging her to sleep. She prayed to keep herself awake. She once said she prayed for the sick two thousand, three thousand times a day.

The heat and fever weakened the sick woman. Annalena wrote that she loved her with an infinite tenderness. Even that love couldn't keep Annalena's eyes open for the nightlong vigil. When her head drooped and her body collapsed in sleep, the woman took the dirty pillow from behind her own head and offered it to Annalena. She was one of the lucky few who had a pillow. Most of the people in the hospital lay on cardboard and used scraps of clothing for pillows. Annalena didn't refuse, though the pillow was full of infection.

Around five o'clock in the morning, Annalena woke, took the woman's hand, and smiled at her.

"Maybe at the end of my life I can say that all I did was pass through this world, holding the hand of the dying, smiling tenderly," she said later.[10]

The light of the kerosene lamp illuminated the woman's face. She fought to speak.

"God is . . . in the name of God, gracious, merciful . . . go!" And she died.

"These people must have an extraordinary reward in heaven," Annalena wrote, "because they have suffered so darkly on earth . . . dead for the mistakes of those who don't know how to treat it."[11]

Annalena started going to the hospital every day. She brought water, eggs, bananas. "Of course," she said, "the biggest temptation is to devote myself entirely to TB, but that remains only a temptation because I am not sufficiently competent."[12]

"In the beginning," Maria Teresa said, "patients treated her like the last thing on earth. 'Annalena bring this, Annalena carry that . . .'" The attitude toward missionaries and aid workers often was, as a priest who spent time in Mogadishu said, "God sent you here to work for us, get on with it." Even secular humanitarians were met with this expectation. Whether it was God or country, someone had sent these people and they should get to work.

Annalena didn't mind. "I can never do great things. I will always do small things. I will be a presence, a witness. . . . We must accept spending our lives not doing anything great or extraordinary. Accept a simple life, trivial, monotonous, understanding that the only valuable thing is our presence. Our coming here is only meaningful to the extent that we are joyfully willing to be manure."[13]

Were small things enough? Like being a presence among the sick? A witness to the dying? Manure? When I moved to Somaliland in 2003, I would have answered with an unequivocal no. I came to Somaliland because of the challenge, because of the bigness of the possibilities. An uncomfortable life in a hard place, a region Americans feared, would increase my chances of greatness. Investing in students who would become the leaders of future generations, breaking down barriers between Christians and Muslims, Americans and Somalis. I would be part of building a nation from the ground up, promoting regional peace.

Annalena saw her role differently. She embraced small successes because she saw each individual as a unique treasure. Jesus said, "What is the kingdom of God like? What shall I compare it to? It is like a mustard seed, which a man took and planted in his garden. It grew and became a tree, and the birds perched in its branches." Annalena understood that this was the nature of the kingdom of God, the way small things multiplied.

Children flocked to Annalena. One boy, Mahamud, had been abandoned in an *aqal* several miles outside Wajir. He was deaf and seven or eight years old. His father had left him months ago and now his brothers, who had returned occasionally to the *aqal* with food and water, left him as well. They had no idea what to do with a child who couldn't hear. He was dangerous. Not that he would harm anyone, though everyone knew stories of men unable to speak or hear who, as they grew stronger, lashed out with their fists or teeth or sharp knives. To keep safe, families chained them to trees or bedposts. No, Mahamud was dangerous because he was a liability, a weakness. He could get lost and make his family lose days hunting for him instead of water. He could catch a disease, and no one would know it and he would pass on the infection. Maybe deafness was contagious. Who could know?

When Annalena found him, he was dirty, starving, and alone. She said he was the most beautiful Somali child she had ever seen.

Mahamud was the first deaf child she took in. He had never been to school but quickly revealed a sharp intelligence. Annalena learned of a school for the deaf in Kerugoya, run by an American named Joe Morrissey. She sent Mahamud there and he performed well in all his studies. During school breaks, he returned to Annalena's home. He would also find a home with Annalena, decades later, in another country.

Many of these children needed physical therapy. Maria Teresa received training in Nairobi and decided to open a physical therapy center to treat victims of polio and other debilitating diseases, accidents, or animal attacks.

A village elder donated twelve acres of land. Annalena drew up building plans, and construction started on the Farah Center, or Center of Joy. When finished, the building was surrounded by a wall and contained several rooms branching off a central courtyard: storage, a kitchen and dining room, a gymnasium with walking machines and parallel bars, staff rooms where the women lived, and a guest house.

"Maria Teresa doesn't like the land," Annalena wrote, "because there are no trees and only a bit of scrub brush undergrowth. Almost too many plants for me, but we both know that Maria Teresa will transform it into a garden."[14] She did. She planted eggplant, tomatoes, watermelon, papaya. An oleander tree grew pink flowers and gave delicious shade. Desert roses, "blood red against white walls danced in the evening breeze." Annalena loved the flat barrenness and mysterious silences of open spaces but admitted that entering the center was like arriving in a green paradise.

Other volunteers joined. There was Lilliana, a nurse who stayed from 1973 to 1981. Maria Assunta Riva joined next, from Cesena, a town near Forlí. She came with Franciscan ideals of poverty, like Annalena and Maria Teresa. Annalena described her as "happy, serene, always singing. She jumps and runs with the children, studies Swahili, and prays a lot."[15] Later she moved to Mozambique, then joined a religious order back in Italy. Linda Pellegrina came; she was born in Kenya, but her family was from northern Italy. Anna Lanzoni, a strict Catholic, helped design and make shoes for people crippled by childhood polio. And there was Inge, a German physiotherapist who introduced "donkey therapy" for the children, teaching them balance and building leg strength by riding donkeys.

Maria Teresa had a motto painted on the side of the Farah Center: DISABILITY IS NOT INABILITY. Once the building and staff team was ready, she brought the people. She found them in huts, in the desert, in town. She joked about bribing the children with sweets to make them endure painful and slow therapy exercises. Then there was Korio, a little boy they nick-named Cigarette.

Annalena urged him to try walking, but he didn't want to. "If you stand up and walk, what do you want me to give you?" she asked.

"A cigarette," he said. She promised. He stood and walked a few steps and Annalena gave him the cigarette.

There was Fatouma, who'd had polio as a child. When Maria Teresa met her, she was fourteen and totally bent down, her head between her legs. Maria Teresa took her to the center and worked with her until she could sit up while tied with cloth to a chair adapted for her. Maria Teresa attached a tray to the chair and if Fatouma balanced her elbows on the tray, "those poor fingers that never made anything" started to make mats.

"She was not so poor after all," Maria Teresa said, "and it made us so happy to see these small fingers working on the mat. She could even earn some shillings and was not as much of a burden on her family."

Maria Teresa put everyone to work who could. Maan, a man with shriveled legs, designed crutches and special boots for the children. Women who could only crawl did housework, cooked, and stoked the fires.

"It was a kind of dignity," Maria Teresa said.

"One day," she told me, joyful nostalgia in her voice, "we were eating. One blind, one deaf, one epileptic, one tuberculosis patient, and us, eating the same food. Annalena said, 'Look, isn't this wonderful? It is what is written in the Gospels, to be among the poor.' We wanted the last ones and we had the last ones."

Not everyone understood, or appreciated, the love the women showed children in Wajir.

Annalena took in another abandoned boy and sent him to madrasa, Koranic school. One day he came home in tears.

"Why are you crying?" Annalena asked him.

"The Master of the Koran says you are going to hell," the boy said.

"But how is this possible?" Annalena asked. "Is God like that? I am here helping people."

"He said if you don't say our prayer, if you don't face toward Mecca when you pray, you'll go to hell." He broke down into harder sobs.

Annalena didn't argue or offer words of comfort. She just let him cry and held him.

One of the first Somali words Annalena and Maria Teresa had learned in Wajir was *galo*, infidel. "We cried when they called us that," Maria Teresa said. "Why did we come here? Because of God – and they call me an infidel. What kind of testimony is that?"

Since the days of the Mad Mullah, there had been rumors in the NFD that white foreigners stole children and converted them to Christianity. Now that there were children in their home, some living there long term, Annalena and Maria Teresa faced deep suspicion from townspeople. Someone decided the best way to protect their children would be to get rid of the outsiders.

In April 1974 Annalena and Maria Teresa walked outside to turn off the new generator that provided lights for the children to study at night. It was late, nine or ten o'clock, and dark. The generator was housed inside a wire cage about eighty yards from the Farah Center. As the women neared it, two men jumped out. One grabbed Maria Teresa, the other Annalena.

Maria Teresa's assailant beat her with wooden sticks that had metal shards on the ends. Over and over, he brought the sticks down on her back, neck, shoulders, and head. The man who took Annalena dragged her into the dirt and pulled at her dress.

Two sounds came at the same time. Someone whistled. Annalena looked at her attacker and quietly said, "Allah."

Both men abruptly ended the attack and fled into the night. Annalena and Maria Teresa stumbled back to the center. Annalena was unharmed but Maria Teresa bled profusely from her head and neck. The children rushed out at the sound of their shouts. Sister Teressana, a Kenyan nun working at the center, stopped Maria Teresa's bleeding and sutured the wounds, but her internal injuries were severe. The next morning, she and Annalena flew to Nairobi where they spent several days in the hospital.

A rumor that Annalena had been raped hangs over this night. Kali, one of the children Annalena had taken in, remembers talk about a rape, but she was a young child and could easily have misconstrued events. A book published in Italy also mentions sexual violence but offers no supporting evidence. As Maria Teresa and Annalena had spoken to no one about the attack, they were shocked to see it reported in this way.

Maria Teresa insisted there had been an attempted rape, but Annalena was spared. She called it "a very big miracle I will never forget."

Maria Teresa had to wear a neck brace for months and still has pain in her upper back. She has a long scar on her head and some limitations in movement. "But we survived. We don't know what they wanted or why they stopped. Maybe it was that whistle, maybe it was Annalena saying, 'Allah.'"

The attackers were never caught.

People were shocked they came back. "But we were so happy to be alive, still with the brains, still with the heart," Maria Teresa said. "We came back rejoicing and singing Psalms 29 and 30."

I will exalt you, Lord,
for you lifted me out of the depths

and did not let my enemies gloat over me.
Lord my God, I called to you for help,
  and you healed me.
You, Lord, brought me up from the realm of the dead;
  you spared me from going down to the pit.
  (Psalm 30:1–3)

"Were you afraid?" I asked.

"No. Annalena was so strong and to be near her . . . I'm not courageous but being near her, you don't feel fear. She was our strength. She didn't know what fear was." In Annalena's letters, I found a quote that helped explain her courage: "We have to be constantly serene and especially when it is hard and smiling takes effort. Otherwise we are outside faith. Either we believe, or we don't. You cannot believe halfway; that does not make sense. So, if I believe, I know God exists and that he loves me and then I am at peace because I accept everything and understand that it is love."

I've often wondered about Annalena's refusal to leave after the attack. Sometimes healing comes not in fleeing the places that break us, but in remaining in them and redeeming them. Every day, as Annalena cared for the abandoned children and the sick, she had to walk past the generator building, past the patch of dirt. By staying, Annalena decided what mattered and what would be remembered. To her, what mattered were the sick and the poor, not her own brokenness. In healing others, Annalena was healing herself.

But the attack seemed to trigger a change in Annalena – an increased commitment to maintaining local culture. A sense that she would have to go much further to convince the community that she wasn't out to remove Somali children from their culture or religion. This may have been what led her to a decision she would come to regret.

6

The Cutting

FIVE YOUNG SOMALI GIRLS lay on their backs on the cement floor in Annalena's compound. The girls, abandoned by their families, had been brought to Annalena, who took on the role of a mother figure to each. A local midwife, Shanqaari, squatted nearby and rhythmically mashed charcoal and *malmal*, myrrh, into a thick, sticky paste. She set the paste aside and turned to the row of girls. One by one, Shanqaari lifted their cotton dresses, forced their legs open, and told them not to scream. Kali, who told the story. Fatou, now dead. Asiya, blind and now mentally unstable. Two more girls, each waiting their turn.

They didn't scream; they were obedient and brave, as they had been trained to be. But they did cry; silent tears trickled over their cheeks. How could they not cry? Shanqaari took a razor blade, a fresh one for each girl, and pinched parts of the girls' bodies they had never shown to anyone before. When she sliced off the clitoris and scraped out the surrounding tender flesh, it was a lightning bolt of pain. By the time Shanqaari applied the charcoal and myrrh paste to stop the bleeding and to hold the lips of the wound together, the girls were faint from agony and the effort of stifling involuntary groans and whimpers.

"Our legs were tied together, here and here," Kali touched just below her hips and her knees, "and the two thumbs," she tapped her heels together, "so we couldn't move. If we needed to walk, we moved like this." She stood and waddled like a penguin, tipping back and forth between the soles her feet with her legs stuck to each other.

For two weeks the girls stayed like this, though they were carried into a private room. Lying on their backs or their sides, healing. It was an appropriate place to heal, the Farah Center, the Center of Joy. This was where these same girls received physical therapy, tuberculosis medications, learned sign language and Braille, studied the Koran, and went to school. This place, where they now lay bleeding, where pieces of their own flesh had been cut out and tossed aside, was Wajir's mecca of hope and healing.

Annalena, whom they called mother, brought food and water, though the girls didn't feel hungry and were afraid to drink too much. Urine was like sulfur on their wounds. When the girls needed to urinate, Annalena or one of her assistants helped them roll onto their side so they could pee into a basin. She then wiped them clean.

Kali was thankful for the company her adoptive sisters provided, and the distraction from the pain. None of the girls hemorrhaged, none developed a fever or an infection. None of the girls died. They were lucky.

"Shanqaari was an expert," Kali said. "She knew what she was doing. And our mother knew to call her." Not a midwife who might use the same blade on all the girls, or her long pinkie fingernail, and thorns to sew the girls up, leaving an opening the size of a sharpened pencil tip. The paste worked well enough; Kali and her sisters are safely sealed. No, Annalena knew the best way to circumcise her daughters.

"Now we understand," Kali said, "that circumcision is dangerous for girls. There is pain for the whole menstrual period, pain when a man comes, pain when delivering a baby. But then? We thought it was good. She thought it was good because she understood Somali culture."

Kali laughed as she talked about her experience with what is now called female genital mutilation (FGM). She was twelve when Shanqaari cut her, or maybe eleven, old enough to have vivid memories of the pain and the aftermath, old enough to know the difference between being able to pee quickly and needing to squeeze out every drop. She knew the pain of her own menses: the cramps, the clots, the battle raging inside her body. But she wasn't angry, and didn't hold this against Annalena.

"It was the culture," she said. "We never talked about it, then or later." It was simply what people did. "I haven't heard of any other Western women who do this to their daughters."

The World Health Organization (WHO) defines female genital mutilation as "all procedures that involve partial or total removal of external female genitalia, or other injury to the female genital organs, for non-medical reasons."

FGM is mostly perpetuated by mothers, often in the belief that it is sanctioned in the Koran. Historically nearly 99 percent of Somali women underwent the procedure, though this statistic is dropping as nations outlaw the practice and anti-FGM campaigns become more widespread, spearheaded by Islamic scholars and influential women.

I struggled with this moment: Kali on the ground being circumcised with Annalena presiding. Annalena was a healer. She loved people to the point of ignoring her own assault in order to stay and serve. She fought for the poor and oppressed and believed in the dignity of human beings created in the image of God. Why would she put girls she called her own daughters through this agony, this physically destructive act? Kali had three ideas. First, at the time, in the 1970s, people didn't talk about the harmful consequences of FGM. They followed custom.

Second, Annalena raised Somali children and kept them in their clothing, their language, their religion. She brought Koranic teachers and had a mosque built on the property. She encouraged the children to fast during Ramadan and to pray regularly. She never attempted to convert them to her faith. Still, some people in Wajir resented her.

And, third, Kali argued that Annalena developed such a single-minded focus on the sick, she couldn't see beyond them. She speculated that Annalena was willing to go to any extreme to maintain her credibility and presence among Somalis. Most likely, she didn't give FGM enough thought to come to this kind of clear-cut conclusion, but with her mind and work elsewhere, she followed custom.

I understood Kali's reasoning. Still, I struggled. Could Annalena really have given less than full consideration to this act, the most controversial thing I could imagine a humanitarian in her context engaging in? I couldn't erase the image of the girls lying on the floor together, Annalena wiping their tears and washing their bodies. How far is too far? It is easy to look back forty years, from a different cultural vantage point, and judge.

We all have secrets. Annalena would carry the secret of her assault to her grave. Somalis in Wajir may have known about it, but there was no reason to publicize anything. She didn't write much about the attack and never spoke publicly about it. People in Wajir also knew what she had done to her daughters; there is little privacy in such a place. But Annalena didn't talk about FGM either, not until her views on the practice changed and she deemed it valuable to be upfront about her earlier participation. Eventually, I would come to admire her even more for that courage and vulnerability. But initially, this event I came to refer to as "The Cutting" stood in stark contrast to Annalena's compassion and love.

The kind of love Annalena lived required deep inner transformation, conversion even. "Here one feels that we are not called to 'convert' anyone but to the most authentic conversion, one that primarily involves ourselves," Annalena wrote. "The conversion to love. Love forgets oneself, one's tastes and desires. The purpose is only to remember the other, their tastes, purposes, desires. Love is never easy. Not loving is infinitely easier."[1]

Love, for Annalena, was always about action. If love were merely feeling, it wouldn't be difficult. Today, I could say I love the poor and send regular tweets about their plight. I could claim love for the enslaved and only buy fair trade coffee. I could cry at World Vision commercials, with their pictures of starving children. But that isn't love and it isn't even compassion. It is pity and a self-serving assuaging of personal responsibility. This is not what Annalena meant by love. She meant action and service to the extent of personally restricting desires and limiting comfort. To love like that requires conversion.

Love like that stemmed from an inner spiritual vitality that began each morning when the women prayed together. Sometimes Annalena read from the Bible, sometimes from the Koran. There were the Psalms, the Gospels, a bit of silence, then simple and sober prayer. No words, until the end, when a few minutes of intercession would be made for the sick, their parents, their friends. Annalena would close, "Sisters, let us start to serve God because up to now, we have done nothing."

Maria Teresa repeated the last line. "Up to now, we have done nothing."

"I brought you something," she told me, when she described these prayer times. She handed me a well-worn book of prayers and Psalms, in English. "I want you to have this," she said. "It was Annalena's. Mostly we read from this book."

I stared at the book. The faded front cover had been taped on several times and the back cover was gone. The edges curled, and the pages were yellowing, some torn. Handwritten notes in miniscule, meticulous writing filled the margins. Some of the notes were on the English words, others marked meaningful phrases. I felt like I shouldn't take it, but I wanted it, badly. I wanted to read Annalena's notes, follow her train of thought, see what prayers touched her. I wanted to run my fingers over her penmanship, like a totem. Maybe some of her faith and courage would rub off on me.

"Take it," Maria Teresa said. "We are all dying now. Someone needs to take these things."

I held the book with both hands. It was so fragile I feared the pages might tear from the binding if I gripped it too tightly. Annalena's prayer book. It felt holy.

I peppered Maria Teresa with questions.

"Why are you asking these things?" she said. "Some of them you ask more than one time."

"To make sure I get things right," I said.

"In that way you are like Annalena," Maria Teresa said.

I wanted to laugh at the absurdity. If only Maria Teresa knew my selfishness, my laziness, the ways I harbored anger, the way I failed to love and serve.

"You want the truth," she said. "And you want to understand things. Annalena was like this."

That much, I could agree with. I wanted to understand. How did love make Annalena forgo extra helpings at mealtimes? How did it help her conquer fear? How did it make her endure terrible heat without complaining? Stay after the attack? Treat people with terrifying, contagious diseases? Cut her daughters? How could she call this love?

How did Annalena maintain faith that God is loving and good in a world filled with suffering and cruelty?

Four hours of sleep, restrictions on food, sharing her bed with sick, homeless children, or with her housemates if a child occupied one of their beds. She lived far from home and didn't go to Italy for holidays, once even going eight years without returning. She endured loneliness, insults, the lack of worldly comforts like electricity and running, temperature-controlled water. She gave up her clothing, her language, the external practice of her faith. And she refused to call this life a sacrifice.

David Livingstone, missionary and explorer in the nineteenth century, said, "It is emphatically no sacrifice. Say rather it is a privilege. Anxiety, sickness, suffering, or danger, now and then, with a foregoing of the common conveniences and charities of this life, may make us pause, and cause the spirit to waver, and the soul to sink; but let this only be for a moment. All these are nothing when compared with the glory which shall be revealed in and for us. I never made a sacrifice."[2]

Not a sacrifice, but rather a privilege. Can this kind of life not be both? Sacrifice and privilege don't need to be juxtaposed. It is a privilege to sacrifice.

Annalena sacrificed, but not in vain. It was not without joy, not without faith. I think she felt the loss of all she left behind, set it beside the thrill of all she found, and was able to render everything sacrificed as rubbish, counting the privilege as gain.

Annalena didn't talk or write about sacrifice and she didn't talk or write much about FGM until decades later. She turned, with all her energy, to tuberculosis.

Amina Dahiye went deaf from measles when she was eight years old. No more education, no more communication. Somali Sign Language didn't exist, and Amina didn't know how to read or write. Her father worked as a consular for the government in Wajir and they were well-off enough to live in a cement house. Of her six brothers and three sisters, she was the one left at home. Amina's family fed and cared for her, though her world remained silent, her days at school over.

Then, Amina started coughing, deep in her chest. Long, uncontrollable wheezing accompanied the coughing fits. A crackling sound followed that she could feel but not hear. She didn't know it yet, but this was tuberculosis talking. Every time she coughed, Amina sent more than three thousand infectious droplets into the air. Direct sunlight killed most of them in less than five minutes but in her dark, unventilated room, the windows pulled shut and covered with thick curtains to keep out dust, the germs lived on. Amina's family encouraged her to spit, to rid her body of the infection.

Amina's cough became increasingly painful and started to produce blood, which Amina would wipe on her hand or dress. She lost her appetite and felt weary deep in her bones. She lacked the energy even to sit up in bed some days.

Already isolated because of her deafness, the cough now marked Amina as dangerous. As one Somali said about this kind of productive, bloody coughing, "The person who is infected with the disease, I will never be close to him, I'm afraid of his air, afraid that his airwave will reach me, or the glass that he drinks, I would have to avoid even touching his glass." Amina's family tried to treat her with injections at the Wajir hospital. The injections affected her limbs. She started to limp and kept right on coughing.

After the discovery of antibiotics to treat TB – streptomycin, then isoniazid and rifampin – medicine flowed into Kenya. But there weren't enough doctors and trained nurses to ensure the medications were properly administered, and drug resistance spread. (Primary drug resistance occurs when someone contracts tuberculosis from a patient who already has resistant disease. Secondary drug resistance can develop when patients don't complete a TB treatment course.)

In 1960, one researcher in Nyeri found "patients without TB being treated for it, those with resistant strains still on their now useless regimen, children under treatment before a proper diagnosis was made."[3] Kenya was in desperate need of cheaper drugs and a shorter treatment cycle, but it was impossible in this context to launch a reliable trial of new drugs or new treatment methods.

Patients defaulting on their treatment remained a major obstacle. Over a ten-year period in one region, out of 5,879 TB patients, clinics lost track of 3,473. Patients left early, didn't take their drugs at the proper times, quit the treatment, and sold the drugs to get money for food. They didn't drink clean water or practice basic hygiene or limit the possibility of contagion within families. They didn't eat nutritious meals. Doctors who recommended these things operated under the naïve assumption that patients had access to clinics, drugs, clean water, individualized housing, and quality food.

In the NFD, where people lived several walking hours from the nearest clinic and where that clinic likely didn't have the right drugs or might be shut down due to staff shortages, where water made people sicker, and where people were chronically undernourished and 80 percent lived below the poverty level, the pressure to provide for their families outweighed the risk. It was hard to see how default or noncompliance could be blamed on the patient. Paul Farmer, an American doctor who works with TB among the world's poorest people in developing countries, describes what was also true among Somalis, "Throughout the world, those least likely to comply are those least likely to be able to comply."[4]

In the twenty-first-century developed world, TB doesn't exist anymore. Or so people think. When cases increased in the United States in 2016 for the first time in decades, when drug-resistant TB started killing people in Minnesota in 2017, when South Korea announced new laws in 2016 requiring every citizen be tested twice in their lifetime for TB, the reports contained elements of shock that this Victorian-era disease was still among us. Paul Farmer put it bluntly when he said, "The 'forgotten plague' was forgotten because it ceased to bother the wealthy."[5]

In an American Experience documentary called *The Forgotten Plague*, writer Andrea Barrett asks the question, "How do we ever live with a contagion in our midst? Someone is sick among us, that person needs care and help, that person is also contagious and can give us what they have. What is the balance between taking care of the community and taking care of the person?"[6]

Tuberculosis may not have been a priority for Western medicine, but it was very much "in the midst" of Somalis. In their huts, their spit, their lungs, their shared meals. It was easily treatable, if people had access to medication and were able to stay in one place long enough to finish the treatment course. The problems Annalena saw in Wajir, from unnecessary deaths to limps like Amina's, compelled her.

In 1974 the Comitato in Italy, comprised solely of her family and friends, agreed to fund Annalena. She would no longer need her teaching salary. She put in her resignation with the Ministry of Education and turned to the hospital. Without any medical training, without an official salary or international organization supporting her, Annalena, a foreign female infidel in the male-dominated world of Somali Muslims, set out to find the elusive solution.

7

The Bismillah Manyatta

BISHAR SURVIVED CHOLERA and hunger, survived polio, survived a crippling leg injury, survived his first fight with tuberculosis, and then died in October 1975, at the age of six.

Asli's husband evicted her from their *aqal* when she started coughing. She wanted to live. She took her child and started walking. They had nowhere to go.

Amina Dahiye's treatment failed. Her family was desperate enough to consider seeking out "white" medicine.

At Wajir's hospital, Annalena oversaw TB medication when nurses failed to regulate it. Friends in Italy sent her books and articles about TB control and combination therapy. She traveled to Spain, then London, to take medical courses. She learned about a recent, experimental exploration of short-course therapy, which could theoretically cut the time of care from eighteen months to six. With a 33 percent success rate, it shouldn't be difficult to do even a little better. Anyone could practice TB control; you didn't need to be a doctor, you only needed access to medication and had to be a good manager. Treatment was simple and straightforward but had to be followed with precision. Annalena could do that.

There was no reason for Amina to limp, Bishar to die, Asli to be abandoned. Annalena could make sure patients took the right pills at the right time and that they stayed in place long enough for an actual cure to take hold. Or, at least she could try. It looked like no one else would.

Before Kenya could actively promote the new short-course treatment, the country needed to run a trial, to make sure patients were actually cured and that the treatment wouldn't contribute to drug resistance.

In April 1976, Annalena proposed to the Kenyan Ministry of Health that she manage a tuberculosis control test project in Wajir. At a global TB conference in Mali that summer, TB control among nomadic populations was highlighted as an urgent priority and Annalena received permission to launch her project, with funding from the WHO and the United Nations High Commissioner for Refugees (UNHCR), to start September 1, 1976.

The Ministry of Health clarified that her project was not a "clinical trial of short-term chemotherapy, it was a practical application of preliminary results of short-term chemo-therapy trials." The ministry also clarified that it didn't have confidence in the project; it was too unlikely that a Somali would stay in place for six months.

Maria Teresa also raised the question of how nomads could be kept in a hospital. Eighteen months? Impossible. But six months? Maybe, just maybe, for a good reason, a nomad could be convinced to stay. But not in a hospital, beneath a roof or inside the prison of four cement walls. Not without their animals or families. Not without some sense of autonomy, dignity, and productivity.

They wouldn't stay for the medicine – that was clear from decades of failure. But if the right context of care could be created, the right combination of medicine and relationship established, a nomad might stay. Annalena had been in Wajir long enough to know what Somalis valued most highly: Islam, community, and independence.

Her idea was to invite nomads to the property around the Farah Center, where they could build their huts on her land. They could bring some of their animals and a family member or two. She would have them sign an agreement that they would not leave until their six months of treatment were completed and their sputum test came back negative. She would oversee every single pill dosage and provide meals. She planned to build a mosque and a school. She would create jobs for patients. Above all, she would know them: their names, their families, their stories. She would listen to their voices and hold their hands and kiss their cheeks, even while they exhaled tuberculosis bacteria. She would tend their wounds and their hearts. If this didn't keep a nomad in one place for six months, nothing would. Could she do it? Would they trust her? And ultimately, would her method be effective?

One of the first things Annalena did was name her project. She didn't use the word tuberculosis – she never would in her centers. She named it the Bismillah Manyatta, two weighty words. *Bismillah* is Arabic for "in the name of Allah." *Manyatta* is a more complicated term.

It literally means "village." But when Kenya gained independence from Britain in 1963, Somalis in the NFD voted overwhelmingly (87 percent) to be included in Somalia, not Kenya. Their wishes were not granted. Soon-to-be-president Jomo Kenyatta said, "If Somalis want to unite with Somalia, they can pack up their camels and go to Somalia." Nearly a decade of guerilla warfare began as Shifta fighters roamed the NFD and attacked polling stations, policemen, and soldiers.

In retaliation for Shifta attacks, Kenyan soldiers rounded up Somali civilians and forced them into one of fifteen different manyattas in the NFD. Barbed wire surrounded these villages. Huts outside the boundary were burned, camels shot, and residents found more than a mile outside were arrested or shot. This essentially made grazing a crime.

Inside the manyattas, life was miserable. Wells and some herds were poisoned. There was inadequate food and water, a lack of schools and health care. Disease spread rapidly. Animals died and pastureland withered. By the time the Shifta conflict ended in 1967, hundreds of thousands of animals were dead and the traditional Somali way of life was severely disrupted.

Despite this, Annalena would take the term *manyatta* and transform it to mean a place of healing, hope, and dignity. She would redeem it.

The first week, only ten patients came to the Bismillah Manyatta. Annalena wasn't allowed to run medical tests herself, but once a person tested positive for TB, the hospital was happy to send them away. The only requirements for entry at the Manyatta were a positive sputum test, to be fifteen years old or older, and to agree to stay for six months. [1]

The sick came with their camels and the canvasses, ropes, and bent sticks for building their huts. Soon dozens were scattered across the sand. There was no real wall, so beyond a small row of trees and a welcome sign, huts expanded outward as more and more people were drawn to the village. [2]

By the second week of her pilot project, Annalena had twenty-one patients. Within six months, she consistently had sixty to seventy.

Each patient was started on the new short-course therapy. A Ministry of Health report on the project said, "All the patients with organisms sensitive to isoniazid and streptomycin were put on daily streptomycin, isoniazid, rifampicin, and ethambutol."[3]

As other doctors had reported, Somalis presented so sick and at such late stages of TB that their dosages had to be adjusted almost weekly as they gained weight from the therapy and the nutritious diet Annalena provided. Once the huts were built, people had slightly more motivation to stay put, but still Annalena had to enforce compliance. Patients signed an agreement to stay at the center and they had to designate a relative who could chase them down if they left early. Beyond this one promise, Annalena put pressure for compliance on herself, rather than on the patient.

Part of this involved directly overseeing the administration of the medications, down to the actual ingestion and swallowing of them. Annalena kept meticulous records, and direct observation became central to her treatment.

People lined up at a table where she set out their pills and small cups of water or the orange drink she despised as too sweet, and her stack of medical charts. One by one, they swallowed the medicine. If someone was too sick to come to the table, she visited their hut. Sometimes she placed the pill on their tongues. She managed these pills around the clock, on a four-hour rotation.

TB pills were large and hard to swallow. If someone refused, Annalena sat with them until they swallowed the medicine. If someone vomited, she brought a glass of water, sometimes a slice of cake to settle the stomach.

"I was with them every day," she said. "I served them on my knees. I was beside them when they were getting worse and did not have anybody to take care of them, to look them in the eyes, to give them strength."[4] Annalena followed the example of Jesus, who never spoke of results. She believed in the power of presence.

The initial project resulted in a 100 percent cure rate among those who completed treatment. Only one patient defaulted, a man who was declared "mentally confused" by the Ministry of Health. He left to pursue treatment from Allah instead.

Eight patients died. Six died before completing treatment, having presented at such late stages of TB they suffered massive hemoptysis, the coughing up of blood. Two completed treatment but died later at home, of other causes, most likely coincidental infective hepatitis. [5]

The deaths devastated Annalena.

The failure to achieve a cure rate this high among Somalis had previously been blamed on what health officials judged as the proud, stubborn, and ignorant character of Somalis. Annalena disagreed and proved they were open to modern health care "on the condition that it wasn't an instrument to control them but something they could control themselves."[6] Allowing them to build their own homes and maintain the semblance of an outdoor lifestyle close to animals was both radical and simple.

"The big idea," Maria Teresa told me, "was not directly observing therapy but to put a nomad in a hut."

"When she did it," Bruno said, "It was all *aqals*. Now they have rectangular cement cubicles. Then, they put up their own hut and when they were cured, they packed it up and took it with them. This is why it didn't matter how much sputum or spit was in there. In twenty-four hours, the sun sterilized everything."

Bruno and Enza visited Wajir in 2012 and found new cement structures. "We didn't know about them before. Now, people spit inside and it stays there; they can't remove the roof. These were built with money donated from Holland. I said, "Who were these silly people who put cubicles instead of huts?" And right in front of me was the lady who did it. So, people try to help but they don't really know what is good."

Besides the sterilization effect, having nomads build their own huts gave them personal investment in their healing and helped them feel more at home, more autonomous and in control. And, keeping people in community had a huge impact on their willingness to stay.

Annalena didn't differentiate between caring for the individual and caring for the community. Historically, before TB medications existed, sick people were gathered in sanatoriums in the misplaced hope that fresh air or total immobilization or a healthy diet would cure them. Though sanatoriums were places of grief and death, they were also places of community. The sick, isolated from the healthy, were not completely alone.

Annalena focused on the whole person. By making the Manyatta a life-giving place, a place of food, spirituality, and education, she made the six months easier to bear.

Some official health reports written by Kenyan TB control specialists at the time of the project got Annalena's hometown wrong, the spelling of her last name wrong, the year of her arrival in Wajir wrong. Someone, probably Bruno, Enza, or Maria Teresa, went through these documents and corrected the mistakes. A dash through the extra "n" in "Tonnelli," a line through "Bologna" and "Forlí" written above it. These were the easy facts, clear details, and even they were muddied by inaccurate record keeping.[7]

Other facts about the project were even fuzzier. Did Annalena invent the manyatta system? Did she develop DOTS, Directly Observed Therapy Short-Course? Did she develop the best cure for tuberculosis, not only for nomads but for everyone?

Some people answered yes to all these questions, but the truth is not so clear. Annalena came decades after the British attempted manyattas in northern Somalia. How was her method different? She came a decade before Karel Styblo formalized DOTS in Tanzania. Why doesn't she get credit?

She demonstrated what would be required of medical professionals to effectively address TB. She set such a high standard that some say her work is impossible to replicate. She is rarely mentioned in academic literature about TB. This lack of mention could be interpreted to mean she left little impact, and at first I found this confusing. The people I spoke with, from former patients to WHO staff and Somali doctors, proclaimed Annalena as the key figure in proving TB could be treated in nomadic populations and in the development of DOTS, which one nurse called "the greatest coup in medical history."

"Did she invent the manyatta system?" I asked Bruno.

"It was her idea," he said. "Invented? I don't know."

"Yes, invented," Maria Teresa said. "To watch the person put the pill in their mouth and to put the nomads in their own hut, in a center."

"She found that giving medicine wasn't curing TB," Bruno said, "because the next day the medicine would be found in the market. So, she thought to give the pills in front of herself. It was just a good idea."

Kitty McKinsey, spokesperson for the UNHCR in Africa, said "She pioneered DOTS, coinciding with new drugs coming on the market, and she observed that one of the reasons TB became so resistant was that people took medications, got a little better, and quit."

"DOTS was her idea," said Miriam Martinelli, a medical professional who worked with Annalena in Somalia, "She started it, yes. She doesn't get credit for it, but it was revolutionary."

Emanuele Capobianco told *The Lancet,* a leading medical journal, "The manyatta system laid the foundation for DOTS strategies now in place around the world." [8]

According to *Discovering Tuberculosis*, Wallace Fox pioneered the use of DOT in the 1950s. And Karel Styblo is credited as the founder of DOTS, adding the short-course therapy to Fox's initial use, in the late 1970s, working in Tanzania.

A formal DOTS program contains five components:

1. Political commitment with increased and sustained funding.
2. Case detection through quality-assured bacteriology.
3. Standardized treatment with supervision and patient support.
4. An effective drug supply and management system.
5. Monitoring and evaluation system and impact measurement.

Fox initiated observing medication intake. Styblo established and formalized these five elements. Annalena demonstrated that without a relationship of trust, without radically caring about the entire context of a patient's care, DOTS would never succeed.

"She was really tough," said Dr. Akihiro Seita, director of the health program of the United Nations Relief and Works Agency for Palestine Refugees in the Near East (UNRWA). "The WHO struggled with how to introduce forcing a patient to take medicine for six months. She was one of the first ones to put it on the ground in a strict way, to literally implement it in full. She was the one who demonstrated that this could be effective."

Dr. Seita explained that in Tanzania patients stayed for two months in a center and then were given a four month supply of medicine to take home. But Annalena insisted on keeping her patients in the Manyatta for the full six months.

"People thought this was too radical," he said, "or that the treatment supervision wasn't supportive, was like a punishment. But the way she managed it was like she was working together *with* the patient. The people admired and respected her."

DOTS would be touted in the 1990s as the solution to the global TB crisis and in 1997 would be accepted by the WHO as the official treatment strategy. And yet by 2006 the WHO would essentialy abandon DOTS as a global solution, at least partly due to an inability to replicate Annalena's intensity of commitment. The system worked but placed a heavy burden on health care workers, who often proved unable to implement it as thoroughly as Annalena did. And what DOTS never included as a main tenet was the one aspect that made Annalena truly successful. She called it love. But it could also be listed as the sixth element of an effective DOTS program: promoting the dignity and complete health of individuals through relationship.

Annalena didn't formalize her work. She didn't write papers or give lectures. She didn't discover new medications. She didn't establish step-by-step plans others could follow. She loved people. She respected her patients. She gave herself away. She focused on relationships, not projects. Though she was effective, these things aren't easily quantifiable and, for better or worse, they aren't how medical aid projects are run or evaluated. She proved Somalis would stay in one location for medical treatment; she proved the financial feasibility of TB control; she demonstrated that strict oversight was essential and possible. But she wasn't a doctor, and therefore the medical world remained largely silent about her involvement.

Though Annalena deserves more widespread recognition, ultimately this silence is probably what she would have wanted.

After the pilot project officially finished, Annalena continued to run the Bismillah Manyatta. The Comitato and the WHO funded the food and medications.

"The project is beautiful and hard together," she wrote. "Sixty to seventy patients for six to twelve months of treatment. Each one is a person for me, an object of thought, care, worry, hope, dreams, joy, and an abyss of suffering."[9]

Annalena had no tuberculosis "suspects," as the health report called them.

"She had Fadouma and Asli and Mohamed," Maria Teresa said.

Still, Annalena referred to TB patients collectively as "scraps of humanity,"[10] a term that at first glance sounds worse than calling them patients. In *Mountains Beyond Mountains*, Tracy Kidder recalled a conversation with Dr. Paul Farmer's coworker, Jim Yong Kim: "Some academic types say to Jim and Paul, why do you call your patients poor people? They don't call themselves poor people." Jim would reply, "Okay. How about soon-dead people?"[11]

Like Jim, Annalena didn't have time or energy for political correctness. Her choice of words – "broken sparrows," "scraps of humanity" – described how the people she loved were seen and treated by the wider world. This was an accurate assessment, especially when viewed through the lens of disease.

Annalena wasn't making a political statement. She was describing what she saw. She was, in the words of Tracy Kidder and Paul Farmer, fighting the long defeat.[12]

"You do things as confidently as possible, you try to win your victories, but you're making common cause with the losers, the poor, the destitute, the vulnerable. So inevitably some of your efforts are going to fail, or maybe most of them, or maybe all of them. But you don't quit because of that, you don't change sides because of that. It points back to why you do what you do in the first place and the answer has got to have something to do with faith and justice."

Maria Teresa referred to that "something" as, "not a call from God, it was a call from humanity."

"What do you mean?" I asked.

Maria Teresa looked at me, clearly pleased. "This should be stressed, the call to humanity. In her letters, Annalena talked about God, God, God. I think she did that just to remind the person reading them how important God is. We never talked about God."

"Never?"

"We knew each other, understood each other. She didn't need to remind me of God. She didn't start from God, she started from the poor and the poor became the thing she wanted to follow, and then God. God and the poor became one thing. For her to help people meant to help God, in the flesh of the poor. In the end, believing in Christ is not believing something out of the world but *in* the world."

Amina's family brought her to Annalena when she was ten years old. She was too young to live at the Manyatta and her family lived in town, so she stayed home but came every day. She sat by Annalena at the pill table and paged through books, not understanding any of the words, while Annalena kept track of the distribution. She took her own red and white pills, not because she thought they would be effective, but because she wanted to please this strange woman.

"People told me Annalena spoke Somali," Amina said, through a Kenyan interpreter for the deaf at the University of Nairobi.

"Did she speak it well?" I asked.

"I don't know," Amina signed. "I'm deaf!"

For two months, Amina came to the Manyatta. But one day another white foreigner came. He had a long white mustache and greeted Amina with a sign he made with his hands. Amina guessed it meant hello. No one had ever spoken to her that way before. She didn't respond but only stared at him.

The man was Joe Morrissey. He and Annalena talked with Amina's parents and convinced them to send Amina to the Kerugoya School for the Deaf. Joe promised to oversee the rest of her TB treatment. Amina was one of the only people Annalena allowed to continue treatment away from the center, but she trusted Joe implicitly. And if Annalena trusted him, Amina and her family did, too. By the time Amina returned to Wajir for the first school break, she was speaking sign language and cured of TB.

Asli, who had been kicked out of her home by her husband, made her way across the desert, fifty miles from Liboj to Wajir. She had heard of this miracle-worker and didn't know if it was a man or a woman. She only knew the name: Annalena.

"All the desert is singing the name," she said.[13] The medicine of this person healed, it was said. It made you forget the nightmare of being shunned and the terror of an evil curse that would never leave the body.

Another man started an even longer walk than Asli, from Uganda. When he arrived in Wajir he didn't know where to go and passed by the hospital. Someone recognized he wasn't local and asked where he was going.

"I have to go to Annalena," he said. "Annalena cures all."[14] Maybe Annalena was a medical center, maybe it was a method of healing, maybe it was a person.

"Annalena is not me," Annalena said. "Most people don't even know me or identify me as a person. Annalena is a symbol, a movement of love, a healing force, and a blessing from God." She and the Bismillah Manyatta had become both brand and myth.

"People attribute miraculous cures to me," Annalena said. "A thousand times my patients repeat that for them in the world there are only two people: Allah and Annalena."[15]

Annalena couldn't cure everyone. After six months of treatment, Asli died. On paper, she should have been fine. Instead, she lay on the ground and struggled for each breath. Annalena squatted beside her and Asli whispered Annalena's name over and over. She pleaded for medicine, her eyes full of pain. She died at seven o'clock in the morning. Annalena was devastated.

People sensed when death was near and called for Annalena. She went to them every time, rushing to meet what she called "immediate needs," no matter what else she was doing. Even when she was praying, she would stop and go to the bedside of the dying.

Annalena once wrote, "I am never so active as when I pray."[16] She could pray in silence, with moans, or with words, but at the same time, prayer was action. Or action was prayer. There was little separation. But for someone so deeply spiritual, how could she simply abandon these prayers?

I asked Maria Teresa and she said, loosely quoting Vincent de Paul, saint of charitable works, "While you are praying, if someone needs you, it is better to go immediately to him because that God you are adoring in your prayer is less tangible than that man who needs you."

It wasn't only death that brought Annalena in an instant. Any need pulled her toward it. Joe Morrissey described a meal at her home: "We were having dinner and the bell rang at the side entrance of the center, at the Beautiful Door. [Annalena called it beautiful because it was where people came to ask for food, medicine, and companionship.] It was a TB patient, weak and with an empty cup in his hands. He asked to be allowed more food. Immediately, Annalena went into the kitchen and filled up the cup with our rice."[17]

Annalena's patience with medical staff wore thin. They didn't enforce her strict direct observation technique; they didn't keep people on schedule; sometimes they took the medicine away and she speculated that it was to be rid of the sick people as soon as possible.

One elderly man named Ahmed came to Annalena, desperate for more antimalarial drugs, which had run out. Annalena suspected he had TB, not malaria, and sent a sputum test to Nairobi. She was correct, though the lab in Wajir had tested him several times and found him negative.

"Assassins!" she said. "They play with human life as you play with pebbles in the sand."[18]

She wrote to Bruno, begging him to come work with her.

He and Enza visited several times. Once, they stayed more than a year.

Despite Annalena's pleas, after the birth of their son, Bruno and Enza decided not to move permanently to Kenya.

"There was a lot of mixing between the sick and the healthy," Bruno told me. "And when I saw my child playing on the ground with someone who had TB . . . I couldn't stand it. I chose my way. It is not a problem; that choice belongs to me." There was a pique in his comment and I wondered if he had struggled with comparing himself to his sister, much as I had, and come up wanting.

I asked Enza. "Oh yes," she said. "I never felt as good as Annalena. But I couldn't live like her."

In the hot seasons, by nine o'clock in the morning, Annalena would feel weak in the legs and struggle to stand. By noon, severe headaches plagued her. Dust stuck to her skin with sweat. The house and the Manyatta reeked of thousands of insects. People would wake in the morning with their bodies speckled with blood from rolling onto the bugs or scratching in their sleep.

"I am ready to bend to the wishes of anyone who is sick," Annalena said, "and give them medicine at midnight if they want, to overcome their initial protests. Some take it every six hours, others every four hours. So, I go to the huts sometimes two or three times a night."

Annalena struggled to find people willing to bring sputum tests to Nairobi to test for multi-drug resistant TB. She didn't trust the lab in Wajir. The hospital had ten Land Rovers, all broken down, and no one would go to Nairobi for parts.

Jealousy hindered her work too. Enza said Annalena had trouble with hospital staff because she wanted them to work like her, even through the night, and they rebelled. They complained she was running a hospital but wasn't a doctor and threatened to force her patients to move back to the hospital. Once Michael Wood of the Flying Doctors flew over Wajir and tried to send a message to "Sister Annalena" via radio, through a doctor at the hospital. "I don't know any Sister Annalena," the doctor said. "I only know a Miss Annalena." He refused to pass on the message.

There were other criticisms. The Ministry of Health mercilessly reported that, "Somalis by nature are lazy and would sit doing nothing except talking the whole day. Their time in the Manyatta could be better utilized."[19] Never mind that many were sick and in pain, or that they attended school and job skills trainings.

Despite the struggles, Annalena was content. "I feel I could die from this point onward – a heart attack, a thief, a military action, a car accident. I could have joy, if not for the violence that often accompanies death, for I have not wasted my life."[20]

She talked often of her own death, with a fondness and a curiosity about what she would find on the other side.

"She wanted to be standing when she died," Maria Teresa told me. "She said, 'Remember, when I die, put me up on my feet. I want to die on my feet.'"

But it was not the time for Annalena to find rest in death. It was time for her to find a partner and a place to restore her soul.

8

Retreat

SIX MONTHS, and Elmi Mohamed would be gone. He hadn't bribed his way out of Wajir, like so many other nurses. He had actually requested a post here. But he didn't intend to stay long, either. Six months was the normal placement for a nurse in a Kenyan tuberculosis ward, and he planned to insist on leaving at the end. Dabar, Elmi's friend and another nurse in Wajir, had asked him to come. Dabar was in the first group of Somali registered nurses to graduate, Elmi in the second. Dabar had already been in Wajir, working with Annalena, for six months and he begged Elmi to replace him.

"I can't wait. I am getting TB every day," he told Elmi. "I have chest pains." He said he was coughing, and constantly worried he had a fever. "There is an angel here, bringing blessing to Wajir." This angel, Dabar said, didn't fear TB, but he remained convinced he would catch it. If Elmi came, *he* could work with Annalena. Dabar could be reassigned to the hospital where TB patients didn't linger.

Patients might think TB was transferred through sex or a head injury or curses, but Elmi knew better. Nurses lived in terror of getting infected. The more one studied TB – how it spread, how it devoured the body from the inside out – the more afraid one became of the disease. An assignment to a TB ward filled with coughing and spitting patients certainly was dangerous. Don't touch the patients, don't sit too close, don't get attached. Do your job and get out. That was what Kenyan nurses were trained to do.

Elmi had family in Wajir, brothers and other relatives from his clan, the Degodia. So he was happy to work there. For a while. For him, returning to Wajir was a relief. He wasn't prepared for it to be a shock.

One of his first days at work, Elmi walked toward the Bismillah Manyatta. He looked at the huts, with people scattered among them, the area free of garbage and scraps.

A woman stood in the middle of a courtyard. He stared. It was Annalena. She held a sick child in her arms "as if he were her own son. She cradled him, caressed him, kissed his dirty forehead, and wiped it clean."

Elmi was stunned. *Never touch the sick, don't get close, minimize contact.* But here was this foreign woman doing exactly the opposite.

"How can a person like her do these things?" he asked himself. "Why her and not me? Why is this white, educated woman, who comes from a rich country where she could have a much better life, doing this for my people who are sick and contagious? And what about me? Why can't I do this?"

In that brief glance, Annalena's influence gripped Elmi. She would have the partner she needed. He soon learned her method of TB control and trusted it completely.

"I was convinced beyond a doubt that she was right," Elmi told me. "But she had problems with the clinical officers. She would tell them what to do and they would say, 'Oh, she is not a doctor.' She couldn't legally prescribe medicine because she wasn't a doctor, so the medical officers had to make the prescriptions. I told them, 'Look, just listen to what she is telling you. She knows.'"

Over the next few months, Annalena's dedication and the absence of fear with which she attended the sick challenged Elmi so deeply that he devoted his life to service in the NFD. He didn't put in for a transfer after six months and continued to work alongside Annalena. The decision would nearly cost him his life.

Annalena walked through the Manyatta during the dark of night. On clear nights, the moon shone bright against the sand. The clarity made everything glisten; she described it as being wrapped in clouds. Patients wrapped in white sheets stretched out on the ground outside where the breeze kept them cool. Sometimes during these walks she heard nothing, no coughing or struggle to breathe, and she rejoiced that the sick had a moment of peace. Then, just before sunrise, she would hear the first of the five daily calls to prayer.

"Allahu Akbar! Allahu Akbar!"

The sick slowly rose. Maria Teresa remembered watching them, knowing they were in agony or feverish. Still, they prayed. They stood and knelt and bowed and each movement brought a spasm of coughing.

"These poor, skeletal sick were able to pray," she told me. "Look how they honor God, while we are in bed. Prayer five times a day is hard, to be so obedient. If I say I learned from a Muslim, people say I am mad. But we really experienced this. Muslims were like a light."

Annalena wrote about the call to prayer, "To many whites or non-Muslims, the muezzin singing is like a scream, terrifyingly scary. To me, it has always been the cry of a man who is not afraid to get up before dawn, to invite other men to stand up and give glory to God."[1]

Annalena provided sticks and saplings and patients constructed a mosque for prayer and teaching. She asked the sheikh, a TB patient, for women to be allowed to pray in the mosque too. He agreed.

"The great adventure of the TB Manyatta was one of love," Annalena said, both her love for the sick and the love she saw in Somalis for God. "People started to say that maybe even we could get into paradise."[2]

Once, the provincial medical officer shouted after Annalena, "This woman is from God! Her skin is white, but her heart is black."[3]

An elder realized that while Annalena provided a place for Muslims to pray, she had no such place of her own. The Catholic diocese in the NFD had a small compound but she didn't have time to walk there. She needed a place near the Farah Center and Bismillah Manyatta. He donated land nearby.

Annalena designed and oversaw the construction of a hermitage where she could retreat for silence and prayer. To get to the hermitage, Annalena had to walk directly past the area where she had been attacked.

A wall topped with broken glass bottles surrounded the simple, square structure. Annalena thought it could be built in a few days, but she wanted a tower, and this caused particular difficulties. There were no two-story buildings in Wajir and there was no scaffolding. Men stacked oil drums, stood on each level, and tossed buckets of cement up to the next-highest perch. Annalena wanted the tower to be several stories high, as close to heaven as possible, but stopped at the third floor. (Maria Teresa thought she had gone too high already.) She put plain, iron rungs in the wall so that one had to climb to the wooden trapdoor at the top. ("Like a monkey," said Maria Teresa.) Through the trapdoor was a small covered terrace from which all Wajir and beyond was visible.

Downstairs was a small chapel with a few mats to spread over the bare sand floor. The Bible rested on a simple table. There was a place to make coffee, and a smaller room for sleeping. There was also a hole-in-the-ground toilet. Everything so a person wouldn't have to leave for days at a time. In the middle was a well with an inscription, the only decoration other than the frangipanis that sprang up later: MY SOUL IS THIRSTY FOR GOD, THE GOD OF MY LIFE.

There was no electrical lighting or water pipes. Annalena said, "Water will be drawn by hand from the well and light will come from the soul."

Annalena dreamed of spending a year in the hermitage. A backlog of work heaped up on her desk. She had so many guests at the Manyatta that she read her Bible and prayed at five o'clock in the morning to avoid interruption. New patients, old patients, hungry children, everyone wanted to see her or ask her for something. Maria Teresa called it a "lacerating dichotomy between silence and the sick. The poor called her back from the hermitage, back to their hell, but she knew it was God who took her to the poor and the poor who took her to God."

She tried to go to the hermitage only when she was sure no one was about to die. People could sense death's nearness, turned their beds to face Mecca, in Saudi Arabia, then called for Annalena.

"They wanted one hand held by the sheikh and one hand held by Annalena," Maria Teresa told me. "The sheikh prayed the Koran and Annalena prayed silently, and together they accompanied the person to the door of eternity. So interesting, that a pure Muslim would want an infidel." She paused. "Maybe no one else is much interested in this, but for me, it is a great testimony."

The hermitage still stands in Wajir, though now it is no longer the tallest building. Weeds have grown up around the well and scraps of garbage pile up in the corners. The Kenyan nuns who work in the Farah Center sometimes come here to pray, but not often. The iron rungs remain firmly implanted in the wall.

Retracing Annalena's footsteps, I scramble up them and perch on the ledge surrounding the small terrace, gazing out over Wajir. Minarets puncture the sky. Camels lumber over dirt trails, led by young herders with sticks slung over their shoulders. The town has expanded and the wells once on the outskirts of town are now in the center. Truckers use generators to pump water and wash their vehicles.

Here, in this place provided by a Muslim for use by Christians, surrounded by stark desert beauty, I feel the possibility of peace, of a world not torn asunder by hatred, fear, and isolationism. The simplicity of the structure speaks of the humility necessary to build such a world. I understand why Annalena lingered here.

She would soon need this retreat even more. One night, after another patient died and Annalena agonized over the lack of pain medications, she went home to prepare a thermos of tea, as she always did, for her watchman, Ahmed.[4] He would come to the door with yesterday's empty thermos and exchange it for the fresh one, along with the set of keys for their new generator.

This night, Ahmed didn't come. Annalena had the tea ready. Ahmed was never late. They had worked together for years and Annalena relied on his trustworthiness, his character, and his physical presence. He used to walk with her to the hospital, back when children threw stones and called her an infidel. He translated for her, able to understand her Somali when others couldn't. She said he cared for the sick and loved them as much as she did, encouraging them and serving when Annalena felt too tired to continue. Tonight, after waiting only two minutes, Annalena started to worry. She ran to the kitchen window and saw the beam of a flashlight flicker inside the generator shed.

"Ahmed!" she called. "Ahmed!"

The light went out and there was silence, no generator rumbling to life, no reply from Ahmed. Dread filled Annalena and she ran from the house. No one was outside. She found Ahmed inside the shed, unconscious, gagged, and bound. He had been savagely beaten on the head. Her call must have scared the assailants away.

Annalena rushed to call Michael Wood of the Flying Doctors, the fastest way to get anyone to medical care in Nairobi. He couldn't fly in at night; the radio beacon in Wajir hadn't functioned in months and strong winds could blow a small plane off course. He flew in the next day and by two in the afternoon, Annalena and Ahmed, now in a coma, were en route to Nairobi. By five o'clock he was admitted to Kenyatta Hospital.

The next morning, Ahmed, the man Annalena "loved most in Wajir," died.

Two days later Annalena flew back to Wajir, lost in her thoughts amid the clouds. "Life continues," she said. "And it takes precedence over pain. But I just want to live in peace. One day all this sorrow and the evil of violence will be unveiled and come to an end."

Maria Teresa said she never heard Annalena ask why: Why is there pain and suffering? Why these people? Why not me? Actually, once, early in her years in Wajir, Annalena wrote down these questions. Then, as she wrote, a peace filled her so deeply that answers weren't as important as her personal response to the pain and suffering. She didn't need to under-stand, she needed to love. She never asked again.

Ruling out random crime, which was rare in Wajir, there were two possible motives for Ahmed's murder. One was to steal the generator or the gas. The second, more likely and with more frightening implications, was related to his Degodia clan association.

Wajir was changing, almost imperceptibly, but small shifts were noticeable to those who paid attention. There were more hungry people, more people from farther away, more crowding around the wells, and more weapons.

Since the Shifta War, the NFD had been awash with weapons. The government urged Somalis to turn in their rifles, but few did. In 1977, Somalia invaded the Ogaden, a Somali-populated region of Ethiopia, hoping to annex this portion of the Horn of Africa that many Somalis believed had been stolen. The war, over in months, was a disaster for Somalia, with devastating consequences for the future of the region. Refugees poured across the border into the NFD, carrying their automatic rifles with them.

Wajir had its own tensions between clans already. Colonial-ists, in a misguided attempt to force peace between factions that seemed in constant conflict, demarcated certain sections of Wajir for certain clans. The Ajuran were given the western portions of Wajir, the Degodia the east. But whenever the rains failed, the Degodia pressed west into what the Ajuran claimed was their territory. By the late 1970s, skirmishes broke out between the Ajuran and the Degodia over water rights, land boundaries, and political power.

As a Degodia clansman working for a high-profile foreigner, Ahmed was a prime target for an attack.

Annalena said Ahmed's death changed her life. "Since he was killed, I am living in a solitude more ferocious than ever. I can't talk about it here in the house; I don't want to cause the others to suffer. I pretend that everything is as before."[5] She tried to rest, to relax, to laugh along with jokes, but the death made everything harder.

"The heat flattens me and dulls the mind," she said. "But that is part of life here and I know in a few months there will be relief. I can't become bitter for all of my sins of omission, but loving is very hard these days."

By the early 1980s, the NFD was the most unstable region of Kenya. Drought returned, and an unbearable heat. Rumors spread of an impending famine. Goats died, people talked about a curse. Shelves emptied. There was no flour, then rice and sugar disappeared. Annalena spent hours moving from shop to shop and friend to friend, to find food. She sent appeals to Nairobi, with no response.

It seemed no one cared about the NFD, or about Somalis, her scraps of humanity. In 1983, Kenyan Minister for Internal Security G. G. Kariuki said, "A good Somali is a dead Somali."[6]

"These are very hard days," Annalena wrote in early 1984. "The generator and windmill are broken; the pump is broken. We have been without water for many days. We draw water by hand from the uncapped wells and are sick. We have incessant discomfort from the heat and the work load."[7]

After writing letters like this, Annalena backpedaled – she didn't want to worry her family. She wrote again, "We have missed nothing. This is the life we have chosen. Nothing forces us to stay, not religious vows, not a religious congregation, nothing. The only reason we are here is love for these people and the love that binds us to each other. We are a happy family, happy women. I am like a mama with her sick children. Don't worry. I have no regret. This is a beautiful life."

Adding to the stress, fresh questions came up about whether Annalena was necessary at the Manyatta. Or, perhaps, too necessary.

A team of anthropologists came to study the Manyatta system. Their primary goal was to solve a new dilemma that had become evident. Could this methodology be effective without Annalena? Annalena found the question preposterous but acknowledged it had already been widely discussed in Nairobi and other parts of Kenya. The same time that the WHO sponsored her TB project back in 1976, they had initiated similar projects in three other villages. None of them succeeded. Kenya still faced a massive TB problem, as did several other African nations and large parts of Asia and South America. Her work was impressive, but was it replicable on a global scale?

This became a consistent criticism as Annalena's work grew in scope and impact. Was she the linchpin and, if so, what would happen in her absence? Was her work sustainable? Could it be formalized? An underlying assumption was, if it isn't sustainable, it isn't valuable.

But if a project is unsustainable in the absence of a person like Annalena, should the criticism be made of her, or of those of us who fail to follow in her footsteps?

"The whole question is one of love and devotion," Annalena said. "But love can't be invented. It must come from God."[8]

This isn't how humanitarians talk. Humanitarians talk about projects and money. Annalena talked about people and love. The sick came to Annalena because they trusted her and knew she would receive them openly with no judgment, coercion, or obligation other than taking their medication. Large, well-funded development organizations flew people into an area devastated by TB, demanded their method be accepted, and flew out again. Or they insisted people follow a program they didn't understand and didn't trust.

Annalena didn't have answers for these organizations about her role or about how to reproduce her work. Until people were willing to embrace Poverty, a word she started capitalizing in her letters, and until they were willing to stay a long time in one place – long enough to earn trust and respect – programs would be meaningless. Long-term solutions required long-term investment.

The issue of whether she was too essential to successful TB treatment, along with the increasing regional violence, sent Annalena to the hermitage. She had profound questions about her future in Wajir and needed to pray.

"I wondered if this was the beginning of a new time, a new chapter in my life with more contemplation and less action," she wrote.[9]

She was wrong.

A surge of violence swept across the NFD. After a series of cattle raids and the burning of huts between rival clans, Benson Kaaria, the provincial commissioner, imposed a curfew on the entire NFD. From seven o'clock in the evening until six o'clock in the morning anyone found outside could be shot.

"The people suffer a lot," Annalena wrote. "By five thirty they begin to close the doors of their stuffy huts – men, women, children, and even goats and roosters. They don't leave a crack. They live in terror. The government has brought a halt to all development in the NFD. We don't know for how long."[10]

Annalena received special permission to move between her house and the Manyatta after curfew, but she begged the local police for a cessation of the curfew, for a return to normal life.

In October 1982 the new district commissioner, Joshua Matui, moved to Wajir. By 1983, he marked a noticeable increase in violence. There were so many dead bodies he was told not to bother sending them to the Wajir Hospital for postmortem exams because it was already known that they had died of gunshot wounds. In November 1983, the Ajuran attacked eighteen Degodia huts. One man was killed and two thousand camels were stolen. A Degodia woman was overheard saying, "The work of the Ajuran will be to bury their dead as long as they continue milking the stolen camels of the Degodia." In retaliation, the Degodia stole a thousand cows, sheep, and goats and killed one Ajuran man and five women.

The year 1984 began with more raids, most often by the Degodia against the Ajuran. Matui's main role was to calm things down. He traveled through the villages urging people to put down their weapons and concentrate on health, education, and development. But he was as powerless as the elders who said, "There will be no more attacks," the day before another attack.

Another goal for Matui was to collect illegal weapons. In December 1983, people were ordered to turn in their weapons by December 26. The Ajuran turned in eleven guns. The Degodia surrendered one. The next day a new deadline was set for January 21, 1984. This time the Ajuran turned in fifteen guns. The Degodia turned in seven.

Neither side was cooperating, but Matui and other security officials blamed the Degodia. Unwilling to acknowledge that no one dared turn in weapons while the other side held theirs, Matui said, "The Degodia appeared completely unconcerned. The Ajuran were being convinced easily by the government to surrender their firearms, unlike the Degodia, who were very difficult."

On February 9, one Ajuran man and six women were killed, and several camels shot in Yukho village. When news of this killing reached a group of government officials having dinner in Garissa, they dispatched a message without interrupting their meal: "All Degodia in Griftu division and adjacent divisions will be rounded up and will be treated mercilessly." [11]

9

Wagalla

"I HAD A DREAM OF HELL," said Father Crispin, the priest for Wajir's Catholic community. "I was standing on a broad plain, before a gate, and there was a curtain across the gate blowing violently in the wind. There was also a terrible confusion of tongues, a babble of incomprehensible languages howling around me. I realized I was at the gate of hell – a strange dream. I did not know then that it was true, that in one week's time hell would overtake us."[1]

In early February 1984, soldiers closed more wells and surrounded others to prevent people from approaching. When a nomadic family came upon a closed well, they assumed the problem was a local malfunction. They took their livestock further into the bush to find water elsewhere. Those wells were also sealed. Degodia men began leaving their families and heading off with their camels. Sometimes they walked twenty to thirty miles a day in a vain search for water. Livestock started to die from thirst and the men grew desperate.

The Degodia have a greeting, "How are things?" The response is, "It's a big world but where I have been, things are fine."

Except things weren't fine. One thousand Degodia men's identity cards were confiscated and destroyed. Camels were found with their limbs shot off. Military vehicles rumbled through town.

On February 10, between two and three o'clock in the morning, Elmi heard an alarm calling all policemen to duty. He was working the night shift at the hospital, right next to the police station. The same night, a military helicopter landed at the Wagalla Airstrip, nine miles away.

Annalena didn't know anything was wrong. By 1984, Maria Teresa had returned to Italy, but Maria Assunta, Linda, and Inge remained. They ran the rehabilitation center and managed food and medicine for the Manyatta. On February 10, Annalena probably woke around four or five and walked through the huts. She would have had a stack of paperwork indicating who needed which pills today.

Before dawn the call to prayer rang out. Members of the Degodia clan performed the Islamic ablutions. *Bismillah al-Rahman, al-Rahiim.* Rinse hands up to the elbow, rinse feet up to mid-calf or knee. Swish water in mouth and spit it out, twist damp fingers inside ears. Snort water and blow nose into the dirt, rinse face. Sprinkle water over the head. In the name of God, the most gracious, the most merciful. They stood facing Mecca, almost straight north.

Kenyan soldiers drove through town. An ominous but not unprecedented presence.

In the Manyatta, Annalena roamed from bed to bed, touching foreheads, asking about symptoms. There seemed to be more soldiers than normal along the roads, but no one suspected anything. Some later speculated that someone performed magic rituals against the Degodia using fingernail clippings or stray strands of hair, or mixed the colors of goats, or used smoke and tea leaves, or chanted curses intended to harm one's enemies.

The violence began in nearby Bulla Jogoo. Soldiers burst into homes and kicked women to the ground. They demanded to know what clan the family belonged to and forced every Degodia male over the age of twelve onto the backs of trucks. The soldiers then descended on those on the roads. Teachers, including headmaster Abdi Sheikh Bahalow; Aabey, a butcher; Matag, a mentally ill man. Men gathered at the mosque for prayers. The soldiers didn't spare the elderly or clergymen. Civil servants on their way to government offices. The next week fifty-two civil servants would be reported delinquent from work. Where had they gone?

After Elmi finished his hospital shift, he started walking home. A large group of men was being loaded onto trucks at the police station, including his brother Hassan Ibrahim Elmi, a retired police officer. He asked why his brother was there but received no response. Elmi's older brother Ugas Ibrahim was also picked up that day. Elmi never saw Ugas again.

The soldiers packed the men into the trucks so tightly that they sat on top of one another, and drove them to the Wagalla airstrip. By the end of the day, between four and five thousand men were crammed onto the strip (though some reports said only one thousand, and the initial government number was 381). The airstrip was relatively new, a mile long, and made of white gravel. A razor-wire fence surrounded the strip and most of the trees had been cut down and hauled away. Heat shimmered up off the gravel in waves, creating a furnace-like atmosphere. The men were given no water or food. They were all from one clan, and with that realization came alarm.

Women and children were left at their huts and animals were left in the bush. When none of their men came back, the women started to look for them. Kenyan soldiers said the men had been taken into the bush and suggested the women accompany them, to bring food and water to their husbands, brothers, fathers, and sons.

Once the soldiers isolated the women in an area called Makaror, they beat and raped them. Old, young, pregnant – they made no distinction. One woman who was nine months pregnant told Kenya's Truth, Justice, and Reconciliation Committee that she gave birth in the desert after being raped several times.

Their huts, filled with all their worldly possessions, were burned to the ground, sometimes with the sick, elderly, or infants still inside.

At the airstrip, the men grew increasingly apprehensive. According to one survivor, a civil servant, the provincial police officer came from Garissa to Wagalla that first evening. He demanded the men turn over their guns.

"What guns?" the civil servant said. "I am a veterinary officer, not a bandit." [2]

"The government is aware that you are here. You are not being held illegally. If you do not cooperate with us, then you may all die here, and no one will mourn. And then we will bring your camels here, and they will die too. After that, your women and children will be brought, and they too will die," the police official said.

Only two guns were recovered over the course of the next three days.

During the night of February 10, the captives were told to lie on their stomachs. Soldiers beat people with belts, guns, machetes, and rocks. Anyone who asked for food or water was attacked. Some captives later admitted to drinking their own urine.

The next day, one man could not bear the thirst and heat and tried to run away. Soldiers shot him, and survivors claimed they overheard them say, *"Hiyo ni nyama ya fisi"* (That's meat for the hyenas).[3] It was the first death at the airstrip.

The men were forced to strip and put their clothes in a heap. This horrified them. These were modest men. No respectable Somali would stand naked in front of another man.

One man voiced the opinion of all. He accused the soldiers of not behaving like human beings. He cursed them and refused to take off his clothes. He said they could shoot him. The soldiers shot him.

The civil servant, who would only be named as F, testified. "They would take thirty or forty men off to the side and light them on fire. You could see the skin burn off them and then they just stood there without skin, their bodies all red. Some of them remained alive that way for several hours. And it went on and on that way, the whole day. . . . We were half out of our minds from thirst and did not know what to think."

In town everyone knew something was going on by this time, but most were paralyzed by fear. Annalena didn't yet grasp the full extent of events, but buried her first dead body, or parts of it, on February 12. One of the disabled patients at the Farah Center had been burned to death in his hut in Bulla Jogoo. She couldn't gather all his remains, because one of his legs had fused to the detritus in the hut. She returned later in the week to bury it there, inside the hut-shaped circle of ash, covering the leg with thorns and stones to keep away vultures.

Acting District Commissioner M. M. Tiema addressed the prisoners. He repeated the demand for the surrender of weapons. Ali Noor, a graduate of Wajir Secondary School, decided perhaps a show of Kenyan patriotism might save them. He started singing the Kenyan national anthem as loudly as he could.

How exactly the next events unfolded depends on who tells the story, but during the national anthem, a stampede began. The captive men surged toward the fence.

The fence was high, topped with barbed wire. Goats and small children had made holes in it along the ground, but not large enough for grown men. They would have to climb or thrust their bodies through the holes. Either way would be painful and there was the risk of a bullet in the back. But a bullet would be preferable to simply standing in line, waiting to be clubbed or burned to death. It was not clear whether Ali Noor started the stampede or whether the men ran en masse, but suddenly the starved, tortured men sprinted for freedom.

The order came to shoot and men began falling. Those too weak to run remained at the airstrip. Those who made it to the fence scrambled over it as quickly as they could. Once in the bushes, the men would be able to evade the soldiers. Most of those who sprinted into the brush were injured, bloodied from the fence or beatings. They were naked and desperately thirsty. Hundreds, some say thousands, escaped.

Elmi, who was waiting for news of his brothers, saw a teacher bring a few injured people to the hospital. He heard a rumor that some of the detainees had been released and thought now was an appropriate time to help, but people told him to leave things alone.

He went to Annalena and told her that people may have been released.

"Let's go," she said.

Annalena and Elmi drove to the airstrip. Soldiers stared at this foreign woman and Somali man. Elmi said they seemed bewildered, as though they couldn't fathom why anyone would drive toward this horror. On their right was a pile of bodies. Elmi watched two naked men carry yet another body to the pile. Water leaked from a bucket and one parched man raced toward the water. Two soldiers beat him and he returned to the rows of despondent men.

The military officer in charge demanded to know what Annalena and Elmi were doing. Elmi was afraid he had endangered Annalena. He said he was a member of the International Red Cross, only a slight exaggeration, as he was a member of the local branch. He hoped that would provide them protection.

"There are injured people at the hospital." He stressed the word injured, as though men were burned and sliced by accident. "They said there are more injured people here. We came to find them."

"We will give you a soldier to accompany you to the hospital," the military officer said. "Those people escaped, and he can make sure they all come back."

Suddenly the soldiers broke out into a loud quarrel. Several cocked their guns, pointed them at Annalena and Elmi, and ordered them to leave. They left, but had seen enough.

When they reached town, someone told Annalena and Elmi that wounded men were roaming the desert. They drove back out to collect people. At first the injured fled at the sound of their vehicle. They came across dozens of women who were carrying water and searching for their loved ones. They found a man sitting in the shade with badly burned legs. They drove him to the hospital. They found dead men still hugging the trees they had tried to hide behind for protection. They searched for hours, until exhaustion drove them to stop and sleep for a few hours.

The next morning, around four o'clock, Elmi's nephew woke him and said his father, Elmi's brother Hassan, had come home. Hassan told Elmi how he had escaped, completely naked. He mentioned a road where other men might be hiding.

Elmi and Annalena painted red crosses on two Toyota pickup trucks and headed to the road Hassan mentioned. Along the way, they found dozens of severely wounded men. They rushed them to the hospital, but with only one male ward, it quickly overflowed. So they carried the rest to the Bismillah Manyatta, the Farah Center, and Annalena's home. Later, the hospital refused to admit the injured, as that would have drawn attention to the numbers. Police cordoned off the hospital to keep victims out.

Elmi heard of another group of survivors near a village called Dela. Again, he and Annalena drove into the desert, along with two more Somalis, Ahmed Jele and Ibrahim Khamisi, and a Norwegian aid worker. They drove through the dirt, to avoid roadblocks, and came to a pile of dead bodies. A military truck passed and the stench that rose from the back made it clear that the truck was filled with decomposing bodies.

By the next day, there were no more living people to be rescued, but bodies were scattered throughout the desert. There was also a frantic attempt to deny what had happened. The Kenyan soldiers had a problem. This was supposed to be a secret operation, but now they had raped women, looted and burned homes, tortured men and shot them in the back. And the victims were loose, running wild and naked through the desert, or dead and rotting out in the open. Or they were in the hospital with severe burns and signs of being beaten repeatedly.

At first Elmi and Annalena buried the dead they found in mass graves in the desert, but then Elmi decided to carry some of the bodies through town as evidence the police would be unable to deny. Sergeant Bashe, a Wajir resident with a pickup, carried loads of bodies, twelve at a time, to the Bismillah

Manyatta, where Annalena buried them in two mass graves. Maria Teresa said that when Annalena returned home at night, she had to shake the maggots off her clothes.

A few days into the military operation, an international delegation from the Red Cross Societies in Switzerland happened to be in Wajir, somehow having gotten through security. They were supposed to visit the local branch but were kept at the district commissioner's office and not allowed to observe anything in town. When Annalena heard they were there, she barged into their meeting.

"People are dying," she said, without preamble. "We need your help."[4]

"That's not true," the district commissioner said. He refused to let them leave the office and forced Annalena out, then told the Red Cross group that she was grossly exaggerating and that they should ignore her. Nancy Caroline, a volunteer with the African Medical and Research Foundation (AMREF) who worked with Michael Wood, wrote, "Annalena did not strike me as the type given to exaggeration."[5]

Because the hospital refused admission, Annalena knew many more would die for lack of care. She convinced the district medical officer to radio AMREF in Nairobi, over a public radio call, a request for enormous quantities of supplies. According to Nancy, at least one request AMREF received asked for fifteen hundred bottles of IV fluid, ten thousand antibiotic capsules, five thousand doses of penicillin, and five thousand syringes.

Nancy was upset with Annalena for making such a dramatic public radio call.

"It was a serious mistake," Nancy told Annalena. "Had the request been more modest we could have filled it without recourse to the Ministry of Health." She went on in her journal,

"Annalena did not see it that way. She had, she felt, won a victory in persuading the district medical officer to radio. What she did not understand was that it was a pyrrhic victory, for it ended up tying our hands, preventing any help at all."[6]

The Ministry of Health told AMREF there was no problem in Wajir that a few ibuprofen tablets couldn't manage.

Somehow, without the Ministry of Health, Annalena scrounged up enough fluids and medicine to treat some men. She lined them up on the ground in the courtyard of the Farah Center. All of them were severely dehydrated and she gave them IV fluids. There were so many, she ran out of places in the wall to hang the IV bags, so she recruited children from the Bismillah Manyatta and her home to come and hold the bags. Then soldiers raided the center. They accused Annalena of harboring the enemy and took away all the men she had gathered. She never heard what became of them.

Despite Nancy's criticism, she took Annalena's plea seriously. AMREF couldn't legally fly to Wajir so she called Mike Harries. Mike was a Kenyan pilot who ran a windmill development project. He had several windmills in Wajir. Thanks to his years of service and his valid purpose for flying to risky locations, Mike possessed what he called a "magic piece of paper." It stated that he was cleared to fly into all remote airstrips, at any time, with no restrictions.

Nancy sounded desperate on the phone and suggested that right now would be a very good time for Mike to "grease the windmills" in Wajir.

Mike agreed. They boxed up supplies and flew to Wajir on February 24. When Mike landed, he pulled out his paper. There was no inspection of his boxes, no questioning, no security detail. They went directly to Annalena's compound. The tension was incredible, Annalena frantic, the people terrified. But she continued to defy orders to stay put and instead buried people and treated the injured.

Nancy wasn't the only critical voice about Annalena's role. Father Crispin told Nancy, "Annalena was too panicky. I tried to calm her, but she would just say, 'I am calm,' while jumping up and down three feet off the ground. . . . If she had been calmer, perhaps she could have done more – and jeopardized less."[7]

Along with breaking curfew and filling her compound with victims, Annalena had photographs taken, which she smuggled out by sewing them into the jeans and shirts of aid workers who were allowed access during the days after the massacre, and she kept a growing list of the dead. Elmi helped her. He asked elders to report anyone missing. At night, under cover of darkness, they matched the names against a list of identity card numbers from an official register. Later the list would be smuggled out, sewn into the trousers of a nurse who went to Nairobi for a training. It included 287 names.

"You should not be making such lists," Father Crispin told her. "We must forget the past. What happened is behind us. We must look to the future."[8] Annalena vehemently disagreed and made no effort to hide her work from the government.

One night she had seventeen Somalis with her to help wrap the bodies they found in sheets, according to Islam, and bury them. One of the men she gave the sheets to, Bishar Ibrahim, was later jailed for fifty-six days. His crime? Working with a foreigner.

Nancy Caroline and Michael Wood mobilized a contingent of people from European countries to visit Wajir, but this was blocked. The lack of emergency supplies led to more deaths.

When people wandered more than half a mile from Wajir, they ran the risk of being shot. When aid organizations were finally allowed back to Wajir, they said they were only there to help victims of drought. Security forces scrutinized every move they made. Any resident caught talking about Wagalla was thrown in jail for six months.

According to an early official report, 378 men were held at the airstrip and released on Tuesday, February 14, having provided no useful security information. There was no mention of finding any guns. Tiema declared the operation a success. G. G. Kariuki acknowledged the destruction of houses and property and admitted that some people had been injured. He also praised the police force for showing restraint while hunting armed bandits.[9]

A newspaper headline shortly after Wagalla read, "Thirteen Killed in Intertribal Feud."[10] As late as August, a Kenyan newspaper reported the Wagalla "incident" as a government peace restoration exercise that ended badly. In truth, the operation had gone massively wrong and now the Kenyan soldiers had to destroy the evidence. The government began a cover-up that would last for decades.

Years later, when the government was finally forced to acknowledge that something had happened in Wajir in 1984, the official number of dead stood at fifty-seven. Residents of Wajir claimed over five thousand men were killed. A clandestine count made by AMREF staff one month after the attack estimated fourteen hundred dead and seven thousand homeless and destitute.

The count was complicated by the destruction of bodies, hyenas and lions ravaging the dead, and grisly efforts of some clansmen to provide semi-honorable burials. The bodies were too heavy and in too severe a state of decomposition to be moved, so people cut off and buried just the heads of their relatives.

In the weeks following the massacre, which many called a genocide, Annalena received strict orders to care only for tuberculosis patients and the disabled. Not widows, not orphans, not the wounded. She must not give out food or help rebuild houses, with the threat that if she failed to comply, her center would be burned down.

"We'll see," she said.

Her compound filled with people who had loaded anything that survived the fires onto donkeys and come to her. They folded their hands and said, "Mungu shauri ya," It is God's will. They came secretly and at night and Annalena wrote down the names they told her of missing loved ones.

"They teach me faith every day," Annalena said.[11]

Eventually she had to turn people away, with tears, as her supplies ran low. "I just put my head down," she said. "The test is immense; there are wounds on all sides."

Nancy brought food and medical aid. She saw both Annalena's faith and her toughness and wrote, "Annalena says grace before meals but there is always a kind of barb in it: 'We thank you, God, for all your blessings, for preventing Mark's plane from landing with supplies, for the food you have given us.' Just a small reminder to Him that His mercy is not quite so infinite as some might wish."[12]

Some of Annalena's nurses turned against her, saying patients had hidden weapons in the Manyatta for years.

"Every act of kindness turned into a criminal act," Nancy Caroline wrote. "When Annalena buried the burned crippled patients, she was accused of establishing an illegal cemetery.

She took local people to help bury the dead and was charged with driving an overloaded vehicle. She took in the wounded, gave IV fluids, kept them alive, and was charged with operating an illegal hospital."

"She was shattered by these accusations," Bruno said. They were excuses, attempts to silence her.

A government commission arrived to investigate. For two hours Annalena told them what she had seen. She described these interrogations as attempts to brainwash her, to convince her that she had seen people dead from hunger or thirst, not beatings, burnings, or bullets.

Someone in the meeting threatened her with death if she went to the foreign press. Someone else threatened to take over the Manyatta and kick her out. In letters to Bruno and Maria Teresa, Annalena insisted that no one publish her stories or go to the press with what she described.

"I certainly don't want to be expelled," she said. "I want to stay here and serve until the end of my life. My hope is that they would rather have me here, even if I am an uncomfortable witness, than have me abroad to reveal all this to the world." [13]

What most infuriated Annalena was that this operation had been planned and enacted by people who called themselves Christians and that Christian leaders in Kenya remained silent.

"Christians who believe they are enlightened," she said. "They raped innocents without provocation, without a war, without personal vendetta. Who did this? A Christian nation? And the cardinal is silent? The bishops are silent? Can we Christians remain silent? I have been arrested, brought before the security forces, interviewed, investigated . . ." [14]

For fifteen years Annalena had been quiet about her faith, trusting her life would be testimony enough. And it had been, to Somali Muslims. But now that Kenyan Christians were interrogating her, she refused to remain silent and spoke out about nonviolence and the love of Jesus every chance she had.

In Nairobi, Michael Wood went to the radio and the press. Then sixteen embassies went to the office of President Moi and protested the massacre. The next week all the leaders who had been involved in the massacre and who were still living and working in Wajir were sent away on compulsory leave. The district commisioner visited the Manyatta and praised Annalena's excellent work. "We are so relieved," Annalena said sarcastically.

Thousands of hungry people came and still those with TB needed her daily. "I feel I will break a leg if I keep walking with them clinging to my hand," Annalena wrote.[15]

Annalena ignored the risks. She had over three hundred women sewing mats to replace the roofs of the burned huts. Despite her efforts, in May, three months after the attacks, much of Bulla Jogoo remained scarred with ashen circles where homes once stood. Father Crispin told Nancy, "Annalena is in grave danger. She has been very foolish, too outspoken. As soon as there is an opportunity, they will attempt to dispose of her, jeopardizing her whole setup. If that is destroyed, she will help no one."[16]

Nancy saw his point, but she also wrote, "There are many things that can corrupt a person, not just money. Silence is one of those things. It is a moral question. A question of the degree to which silence makes you an accomplice to a crime."

Annalena was not one to remain silent. "I am an uncomfortable witness," she said, "beloved by the people, an immense nuisance to the authorities."[17]

Eighteen months after the massacre, in August 1985, Annalena's work permit needed to be renewed. Her request was denied. She was forced to leave within forty-eight hours. Elmi drove her to the airport. Annalena seemed upset, but calm. There was nothing she could do, not even when the man who stamped her paperwork with the blacklisted "persona non grata" thanked her for all the work she had done for his people.

She said the Bismillah Manyatta had been the greatest adventure of her life. Now, after sixteen years in Kenya, the adventure seemed over.

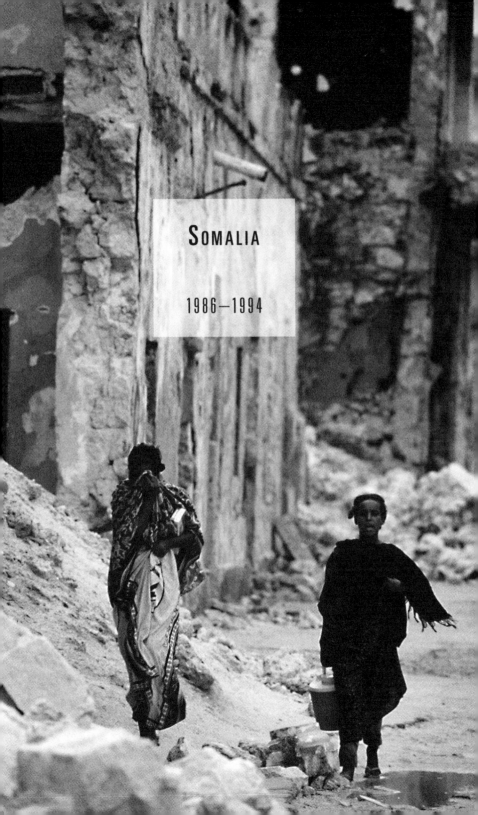

SOMALIA

1986—1994

10

Beledweyne

"DID ANNALENA CHANGE after Wagalla?" I asked Maria Teresa.

"I don't know," she said. "But she never stopped talking about the poor." Not even while she was in Italy. Once, Annalena spoke to a group of young people and said, "To love the poor (and you must remove the word 'poor') means to love a single person. It is to be near, to listen, to try to understand. All people inside are infinitely beautiful and at the same time, horrifying."[1]

Her family hoped she would stay in Italy. Even if she sequestered herself in hermitages, she would be safe and nearby. Surely sixteen years in Africa was enough. But Annalena couldn't adapt to Italian life, a life she saw as rife with hypocrisy and complacency. She had little patience for questions like the one another group asked, "How many camels are you worth?"

She secluded herself in Cerbaiolo and Monteveglio, Franciscan hermitages tucked into cliffs overlooking dense forests. She rejoiced when there was so much snow people couldn't make the drive to visit. The only significant amount of time she spent with her family was when her father was dying. In January 1986, she was grateful to be at his bedside as he breathed his last. After that, her longing to return to the desert became irresistible.

"Somalis are only trouble for you," Elmi told her, and urged her to go somewhere else. But on December 14, 1986, Annalena flew from Rome to Mogadishu, Somalia.

Beledweyne is 212 miles from Mogadishu and one paved road runs between the cities. During the 1980s, this farming region saw an influx of refugees fleeing the disastrous war in the Ogaden. The war had been President Siad Barre's attempt to win one of the five divided Somali-populated regions in the Horn of Africa. But the war turned into an economic and humanitarian crisis for Somalia. Refugees settled in camps around Beledweyne. There was no tuberculosis control and the disease spread rapidly in the close quarters of the camps. One small hospital served the city, staffed by Somalis and Italians.

Miriam Martinelli received two pieces of advice during her orientation to Somalia in the late 1980s. First: no visitors. It wasn't safe. Miriam found this disconcerting. If Somalia wasn't safe enough for visitors, how was it safe enough for long-term staff?

"But at that time, we weren't afraid of everything," she said. "We didn't have the internet or cell phones or news reports. People had guns, there was some unrest, but none of it was affecting humanitarians. It was between Somalis. No one could imagine what Somalia would become."

The second piece of advice at Miriam's orientation: if someone asked for her car, the correct response was, "Here are the keys." With that extensive preparation, the Italian Medical Team sent her to Beledweyne.

"The car advice was because of me," Antonio Gabrielli said. Antonio and I perched on bar stools at an outdoor café in

Pordenone, Italy. "The fighting then, yes, it was there, but not against us. It was revenge between families."

Trim and graying, Antonio now worked in health care administration. He had been the first member of the Italian Medical Team to be carjacked in Beledweyne. He drove up to his house one evening before Miriam arrived, and three or four people waited for him at the gate. When he stopped to give the guard time to open the gate, one of the strangers pulled out a gun.

The muggers ordered him out of the car and pushed him with the gun into a cowering position. He was certain they were about to kill him. His own guard had no weapon. Instead, they drove away with the car. But after that all the foreigners were forced to live at one compound.

All except Annalena.

For the first time in her life, Annalena had a contract and a salary for her TB work. The Italian Corporation paid her to develop TB control in Beledweyne. She worked alongside members of the Italian Medical Team, including Antonio and Miriam.

"It was a lot of money," Antonio said. "And you know what she was doing with it? Not keeping it. Absolutely not. She used it for food and medicines."

Antonio described her house as a stick hut; Annalena called it a shack with a tin roof. A photograph shows Annalena in front of the southern Somali house, made of sticks with grass spread over the roof and a *loox*, a long narrow piece of wood used for Koranic lessons, leaning against the wall. There is a *fadhi*, a four-legged stool with a piece of hide for the seat, and a *gilgirid*, an incense burner. In one letter, Annalena said she found it charming and private, but in another she complained she couldn't work at home because of the lack of privacy.

"I pay the consequences," she wrote, of choosing to live among the people.[2] The heat inside her "oven" house was oppressive, but she preferred it to living at the Italian compound, where the houses were mansions by comparison and would wall her in, away from Somalis. Plus, through gaps in the tin roof and stick walls, she could see acacia trees, foliage, and the moon and stars. Even as she slept on a thin wooden board, she felt like a queen.

I asked Miriam if anyone was jealous of Annalena's freedom and autonomy. The question felt natural, but later I realized it was not the normal follow-up question. The question should have been, "Was anyone upset that Annalena took such risks, potentially endangering everyone else along with herself?" This is what people usually ask about intrepid journalists and aid workers.

What were they doing there, in this place they weren't "supposed" to be? Why did Amanda Lindhout, the author of *A House in the Sky*, which describes her 460 days of captivity in Somalia, go to Mogadishu in the first place? Why didn't Paul and Rachel Chandler, held hostage by pirates, consider their proximity to Somalia when they went sailing? The unspoken implication is that these victims are foolhardy, and somehow complicit in or responsible for their subsequent traumas.

But I didn't question the wisdom, risk, or impact on others of Annalena's choice. In asking Miriam about envy, I had to ask myself the same question. I came to Somalia thinking I wanted to live like Annalena did: an outsider, but adapted as much as possible. I discovered I didn't really want to live that way; I wanted to be *known* as a person who lived that way. I wanted the accolades that come in some circles, especially religious circles, from "going local." I didn't want the cultural stripping or the physical challenges that would be required of me.

Antonio was the district medical officer in Beledweyne and when I asked him a similar question, he said, "Some people feel a challenge when they see Annalena's life and then they can't do it. There can be complicated feelings."

"Everyone assumed we were there for money," Antonio said. "But it was clear she was there to help people. No one tried to rob her; they knew she had no money. Muslims defended her; it was like nobody was allowed to touch her."

Miriam said no one on the Italian Medical Team envied Annalena's freedom or lifestyle. "There wasn't anything to do at night anyway," she said. "No disco or cinema. Not even any alcohol, unless it was shipped in from Mogadishu or created from denatured alcohol in the clinic." She laughed. "This only gave us a big headache."

"Sometimes she came to eat spaghetti with us." Antonio said she drove herself, alone in her gray Fiat Campagnolo. "We played music, we danced. She liked to come. Of course, she would only eat two spaghetti noodles, nothing more. You cannot imagine her taking a big scoop." He acted out plucking two thin noodles from our plate of appetizers. "She didn't drink, maybe a Coke but no beer, but she laughed at us."

Heat and insects defined much of expatriate life in Beledweyne. Annalena battled mosquitoes, comparing their noise to airplanes, and flies swarmed her eyes and mouth while she wrote letters. Pediatrician Mario Neri, who would later join Annalena, made a list of what kept him awake: cockroaches, grasshoppers, crickets, spiders, praying mantises, geckos, mosquitoes. He heard every scamper of rats across the roof and scorpions brushing against the tin cans that covered the legs of his bed to keep them from climbing up.

"Once, there was a cricket invasion," Miriam said. "The air was full of the little black beasts, so many that we couldn't even open the door." To get rid of the infestation, they poured kerosene everywhere: on the floor, the walls, plants, furniture. The crickets looped as though they were drunk or dizzy, then the Italians lit them on fire. "Oh, then we had a mountain of grilled crickets. They smelled so good, like shrimp."

The cricket invasion happened while Annalena lived in Beledweyne, but she didn't write about it. Her letters consisted primarily of work, perhaps one sign of how she changed after Wagalla. It was easy to imagine that, had there been a cricket infestation in Wajir, she would have taken delight in the "little black beasts." I can picture her laughing about the swarms, even as they drove her mad and distracted her from her work.

"One of my colleagues joked (but was it really a joke?) that I am only happy between spitting TB patients, lepers, and the poor," she wrote.[3]

Annalena started with forty-five tuberculosis inpatients and one hundred and five outpatients. Only the very sickest stayed in the hospital. Her first complaints, as they had been in Kenya, were about the medical staff.

"Staff are absolutely not suitable at the TB center," she wrote. "You cannot leave them with written instruction on treatment and observation because they read with difficulty and have never been to school. They are outrageously dishonest from a professional point of view – no dates or wrong dates marked on therapy. They act innocent when confronted. Human life counts for nothing."[4]

Traders – men with no medical knowledge – ran the pharmacies. They sold medicines stocked alongside food and clothes, including antibiotics and tuberculosis medicine.

Annalena remained uncompromising in her standards. Diagnosis was the easy part. Again, people presented at such late stages, many were already coughing up blood. She didn't need an X-ray machine, which she didn't have, and could rely solely on sputum tests.

She said to Antonio, "Come on. If a man is coughing for six months, very thin, very weak, with blood in his sputum, what can I do? It is TB."

Word of a healer spread throughout the region.

Abdoulqadir, who goes by Shaatos, heard of this foreign healer. He grew up in the Hiran region and had known all his life that the most common way of getting *qufac* was either from a curse or through heredity. Shaatos also knew medicine had little to do with healing *qufac*. The first method, burning the sick with coal or ash, corresponded to the Somali proverb, *Dab iyo cudur meel ma wada galaan,* "disease and fire can't exist in the same place."

The second method was smoke. The coughing person leaned over a fire with a blanket draped over his or her head and shoulders, to inhale the smoke. This was most effective if a spirit caused the cough because the smoke, and the accompanying dances of the men and women who watched, chased away the evil spirit.

But Shaatos heard of this woman who had other ideas about disease and healing, and he went to Beledweyne to find out more.

After orientation, Annalena weighed patients and started them on treatment. She still counted every pill and watched it be swallowed. Those who signed the contract and swallowed their pills felt better within two weeks. Her big challenge then was to convince them to stay for six months, to wait for the complete cure. One patient wanted a week's supply of TB drugs so he could take his flocks to pasture; she refused to give it and refused to let him leave.

"She was ready to fight," Antonio said, to keep them in treatment. "She could force them, and they listened to her. She was small but not weak. Fierce. Respected. But not in a white, colonialist way. She got angry if they didn't take the medicine in front of her, but it was an anger that wasn't offensive. They could tell she wanted the best for them."

She wrote, "They call me a *waddada*, a holy woman. A person of miracles, a place where someone cares."[5] Though she would deny performing miracles, I like this image of Annalena as both person and place. Aid workers who drop in and run away at the first sign of trouble, or at the end of impossibly brief contracts, can't offer the stability Annalena did that led to her being referred to as a place. But I was also curious about her perception of her spiritual role, how she felt about being called a holy woman.

Carlo, another member of the Italian Medical Team, and one of the most beloved surgeons in Beledweyne, was the first person I spoke with to call Annalena a saint.

I asked Bruno if Annalena was a missionary. He didn't answer.

"Catholic? Christian?"

No answer. After a long pause, he said, "Annalena hated when people called her a missionary. She said she was consecrated to the poor and to God, through the poor. She refused labels."

Maria Teresa didn't answer right away either. "She loved Jesus and tried to follow his teachings. She said 'Allah' for God. She read Hindu teachings. She loved people, these other things don't matter. That is the lesson of Annalena."

Annalena undeniably followed Catholic traditions in her own practice of faith, mostly in the privacy of her home, though on the few occasions she was in Mogadishu, she attended Mass at the cathedral, led by Bishop Salvatore

Colombo. The Mogadishu Cathedral was where she met Father Giorgio Bertini.

Because she lived so far from the cathedral and from other practicing Catholics, the bishop granted Annalena special permission to keep in her possession the Blessed Sacrament. Father Giorgio gave it to her.

"But where will I keep it?" she asked him.

"Don't worry," he said, "you'll know where to put it."

"I did not ask for it," she wrote. "I don't have a safe place to keep it. But the important thing is that the Lord has returned to Beledweyne after so many years." Annalena wrote of two specific things bringing life into the loneliness in which she found herself throughout the years: having the Eucharist in her possession, and the success of starting Koranic schools where Somalis with TB could learn and grow in their faith.

That Annalena would equate the bread with the presence of the Lord struck me as the single most Catholic thing about her.

Father Giorgio concurred. After clarifying for me the Catholic belief in transubstantiation, in which the bread becomes physically and literally the body of Jesus, he added, "The body of Christ is present as long as the bread is. It must be renewed. If the elements become corrupt, the body of Jesus is no longer there. There is the need to constantly eat it and replace it. Corruption could come from humidity, or ants."

There, in a stick hut, surrounded by Muslims, in the middle of a brewing civil war, Annalena would safeguard the body of Jesus.

"The Eucharist is scandalous to atheists and other faiths," Annalena said later in a speech. "It contains a revolutionary message: 'This is my body, made into bread so that you, too, can be bread at the table of humankind, because if you don't make yourself bread, you don't eat the bread that saves but you eat to your own condemnation.' The Eucharist tells us that our religion is futile without mercy. In mercy, heaven meets the earth."[6]

Annalena's faith confused many people.

"She said Allah for God," Antonio said. "This was radical for a Catholic. She didn't want to convert anyone, though. She said, 'What's the difference?'"

"She had been rejected by the Catholic community," Miriam said, and talked about the lack of support, financial or physical, from the Catholic Church. "That she continued to read her Bible – I couldn't understand this."

"I never understood her motivations," Antonio said. "Why was she there? Of course, faith, but . . . I've thought a lot about this. I don't understand."

Annalena wasn't oblivious to the way her radical faith flabbergasted people. "I don't even try to be understood in my desire to serve, to just wash feet," she wrote. "I'll accept misunderstanding to the end of my days. No one agrees even in part with my choices. But there is less criticism, less rebellion. Admiration and respect have taken over. Italians and Somalis call me *hooyo*."[7]

A few years later, people like Annalena would earn another nickname, this one derogatory: White Saviors. And their work would be described as a complex, loaded with elitism, privilege, racism, and the promotion of a colonialist mentality.

In *The Road to Hell*, about humanitarian aid, mostly in Somalia, Michael Maren wrote, "We all just knew, somehow, that our breeding, education, and nationality had imbued us with something valuable from which these less fortunate people could benefit."[8] The term "white savior complex" hadn't been coined at the time Maren wrote this, or when Annalena lived in the Horn, but this is the conceit: the white, Western volunteer or employee carries an innate ability to save the desperate, poor, abandoned African.

This stereotype is perpetuated by movies like *The Blind Side*, in which the poor black boy is taken in by a wealthy white family, or *Freedom Writers*, in which the white teacher becomes the creative hero saving her black students. Teju Cole wrote in his article "The White Savior Industrial Complex," published in the *Atlantic*, "The White Savior Industrial Complex is not about justice. It is about having a big emotional experience that validates privilege."[9]

In these scenarios, the desire of the foreigner to serve takes precedence over best practice and the foreigner is the one who gets to define that service.

Where does Annalena fit into this narrative? Cole writes: "There is the principle of first do no harm. There is the idea that those who are being helped ought to be consulted over the matters that concern them." That was a starting point for Annalena. Tuberculosis needed to be treated, the Kenyan government asked her to run their project, and she consistently made agreements with local Somali authorities to ensure she was doing work they wanted and valued. Also, TB launched her into a lifetime commitment – not a few months or even a few years, but decades of caring for the sick.

"Everyone was thinking she suffered from this complex," Antonio said. He meant not that she had a hero complex, but that she was too invested. She couldn't see herself as separate from the people she helped, which was a principal tenant for aid workers. Ostensibly, this was to maintain objectivity, but objectivity was never Annalena's goal.

Antonio said she provided the best TB control anywhere at that time. Carlo said the World Health Organization would have had to hire one hundred people to do the work she did. Still, criticism came from the medical establishment. She wasn't a doctor, and never claimed to be one, and doctors looked down on her. The authorities resented her projects because her humility, consistency, and success exposed their weaknesses. They complained that her method required someone be available to do follow-up appointments, to be at the clinic every day, to see every patient. They complained she was too popular and couldn't tell the difference between private life and work life.

Experts criticized her for caring too much. She criticized them for not caring enough.

"If someone wants to come," she said, in response to complaints that no one would continue her intense style of work, "and do this work differently or learn about it, they can come." But no one came.

"She suffered from this disease [the white savior complex] if we can call it a disease," Antonio said. "She said, 'If I don't help them, they will die.' So, she did save people, that is true. Some say let them die. But she tried to help."

Miriam Martinelli said, "It was the 80s, 90s. People were dying. We tried to help. No one talked about these things at that time."

While Miriam's words are true, they are not a sufficient excuse. It is precisely the mishandling of aid work through these decades that contributed to the problem of the white savior. But this idea of Annalena herself having a white savior attitude "was more an issue for those criticizing, less for Somalis," Miriam said.

I asked Bishop Giorgio. "I would say, yes, she was a white savior. But she was doing it for the abandoned. Yes, she was a bit dictatorial and too white, but I would still support her. She was serving, not living a luxurious life. That is the best answer. She committed her life while others just look and criticize."

This is the crux. She committed her entire life. She did not become wealthy or famous; she didn't seek her own comfort or safety. She never used her skin color or privileged background for personal gain. She trained local nurses and partnered with Somali physicians. Westerners questioned even this practice, saying she failed to train a successor. While she didn't explicitly say so, I believe she expected Somalis to be her successors, and they have been.

To label her a white savior and say she should never have gone to Kenya or Somalia can't be the right answer. The white savior complex is bestowed on people like Annalena by outsiders who lump all foreign aid workers into the same category. There are certainly examples of aid workers with this attitude, but Somalis who knew her rejected the term.

Elmi said Kenyan Somalis would never say Annalena suffered from a hero complex. He agreed with Bishop Giorgio, that the people who most took issue with her work were those who stood by and observed, quick to criticize and slow to sacrifice their own positions of privilege and power.

In Beledweyne "the heat blunts everything," Annalena wrote.[10]

She found mental relief in focusing on the poetic nature of the desert. At night the stars were so bright she described them as living next door and said the dusty sunsets over palm trees were straight out of *Le Petit Prince*.

When rain came, patients emerged from their huts, some of them wearing only underwear or loin cloths, and lifted their faces to the sky to feel the cooling rain on their feverish skin. The dust washed away and even patients too sick to stand crawled outside, their bodies shaking from disease and excitement about the rain. One man leaned on his walking stick and bowed his head, a small, private smile on his face.

But the rain didn't stop. The Shebelle River, which snakes through Beledweyne, rose. In June it flooded over the embankment. Annalena needed to evacuate the tuberculosis patients, but higher, drier ground was on the other side of the river and the only way across without going miles out of the way was on a raft that two men steered using a pulley system. The higher the river rose, the stronger the current became, and the more dangerous the crossing.

Annalena loaded seven or eight people at a time onto the rubber raft, along with medications, folders, mattresses, and household supplies. She started with the sickest, those who were bedridden and closest to dying. Once they were all across, she moved them into three rooms at the Beledweyne hospital.

"The healthy people," those without tuberculosis, "were horrified. They didn't want my sick and poor." Annalena hoped life would normalize soon. She didn't love these adventures – they stole her already limited opportunities for solitude and prayer. "I am unquenched in my desire for silence at the feet of God," she wrote in the middle of the flood crisis.

She didn't move across the river, despite the Italian Medical Team's insistence she move into their compound. One of the doctors asked what she would do when her house flooded. The water was already at the brink of her compound.

"I will sit on top of one of the big trees in my backyard," she wrote.[11]

Interfamily revenge murders, drought, and flooding were not the only security concerns around Beledweyne in 1987.

Somaliland, in the north, had gained independence from Britain on June 26, 1960. On July 1 that same year, southern Somalia was released from Italian administration. Seven months later, on January 31, 1961, the Somalia National Assembly proclaimed a new act of union for the north and the south. The act was drafted by southern Somalis and Italians; Somalilanders were not allowed to make changes to the document and the union started off with a clear delineation between north and south. Initially, both north and south were euphoric, hopeful that the NFD in Kenya, the Ogaden in Ethiopia, and Djibouti, which had been colonized by France, would also soon be united. This hope, which has still not been realized, is symbolized in Somalia's flag: a white, five-pointed star against a blue background.

It quickly became clear that with the government located in the south, far from northern interest and pressure, rule would not be balanced. Less than a year after the act of union passed, Somaliland military officers unsuccessfully attempted a coup against the southern government. A precarious peace followed.

Somalia's first president, Abdirashid Ali Sharmarkey, was assassinated in October 1969 and Siad Barre took charge. Barre publicly denounced clan allegiances. One of his well-known sayings is: "Tribalism and nationalism cannot go hand in hand. It is unfortunate that our nation is rather too clannish; if all Somalis are to go to hell, tribalism will be their vehicle to reach there." But, in private, Barre manipulated clan loyalty and systematically placed members of his own clan, the Darood, in positions of government authority.

Barre's stranglehold on Somalia tightened after the failed Ogaden war. Now that Somalis of every clan were armed, thanks to Soviet and American weapons, Barre needed to tamp down all forms of dissent. In 1988 he launched a brutal attack against an Isaq clan rebel group in Hargeisa, the capital of the north. Some said as many as fifty thousand Somalis were killed by warplanes that took off from their own airport, bombed by their own president.

The massacre was one more step on the path to civil war, which would reach Beledweyne soon.

Italians built the Mogadishu Cathedral in 1928. It was stunning, with arches, pillars, and bell towers that gave it a Gothic flavor. Scenes of prophets, disciples, and saints decorated the walls. One, of Francis of Assisi with two sheep, would later become a shooting target until Francis's face was completely destroyed. Now, in the 1980s, it served a Catholic population of a few hundred Somalis and over a thousand Italians.

At 7:15 p.m. on Sunday, July 9, 1989, after Mass, Bishop Salvatore Colombo walked through the cathedral courtyard. Earlier that day, a man had asked Bishop Colombo for an interview. After Mass the same man approached, raised a gun, and, at close range, fired a single shot into the bishop's chest. Bishop Colombo died at the hospital.

No one claimed responsibility for his assassination. Speculation fingered the president, since the bishop had been an outspoken critic of his regime. Barre blamed Islamic fundamentalists.

Five days later, after Friday prayers, the citizens of Mogadishu staged a massive anti-government demonstration. Soldiers opened fire and killed hundreds of people. Thousands more were arrested. Forty-six of them were lined up on Lido Beach and shot by firing squad. The country descended into chaos.

11

Hostage

ONE BY ONE, aid organizations abandoned Beledweyne. Save the Children, Eastbrook Church, and Swedish Church Relief left. Of the foreigners, only Annalena and the Italian Medical Team remained.

In December, rebels robbed the head of UNHCR in the nearby village of Jalalaqsi. The last UNHCR car in Beledweyne was stolen. Then armed rebels took the bus that ferried people to Mogadishu. Annalena finally acknowledged that the country was at war, "but we are still alive." The conflict felt specific to Somali grievances with the government and it was hard to see how foreigners would be affected, as long as they could avoid stray bullets and maintain a supply of food and medicines.

"It is true," Annalena wrote to her mother, "the situation is not quiet. But where is there calm and peace in Africa? In the world? I am fine." [1]

In July, cannons exploded all around Beledweyne. None of the Italians slept the night of that first serious attack. Miriam and Carlo remember diving under their beds for safety. Antonio played cards at the IMT compound with Elio and Rosa, other members of the IMT. They tried to keep the game going, to pretend things were normal and safe but eventually they, too, ducked beneath the table.

Annalena's home was unguarded, without a security wall. But she didn't hide and didn't confess fear. She said her house was probably the only place in the village where people could feel relaxed and calm.

In Wajir, Annalena had faced danger a couple of times. Now, however, and for the rest of her life, facing guns, threats, and violence would be a near-daily occurrence. She showed a courage hardly possible for organizations or governments. If the first priority is sustaining an organization, when trouble comes humanitarians flee. Right when the needs become urgent, people are abandoned.

"I can't even think of the cannon or the machine guns," she said. "I am too full of the sick, the suffering, and Jesus Christ. It is as if I am in another world." [2]

The next day Miriam and one of the lab technicians left Beledweyne for Mogadishu. The Italian embassy radioed and ordered the rest of the IMT to evacuate to Jalalaqsi. They believed rebel fighters were circling and closing in on Beledweyne. The team would be safer in Jalalaqsi.

This time, Annalena came along when the IMT invited her. She had often talked of her willingness to die alongside Somalis. She told Antonio she dreamed of one day dying as a martyr. The comment would have made most people sound slightly insane, but from Annalena, Antonio accepted it as a simple and natural expression of her faith and lack of fear. So why she moved to Jalalaqsi with the five other Italians isn't entirely clear.

Antonio thought she made a wise decision. She talked with him about the privilege of death, and could be stubborn, but she wasn't foolish. "People there have tuberculosis too," she told him. "I can work there." She told her TB patients in Beledweyne to follow her to Jalalaqsi, and they did.

Three days after the move, around three in the afternoon on August 25, 1990, rebel fighters descended on Jalalaqsi.

Antonio and Carlo were at the hospital when the shooting started. Annalena, Elio, Rosa, Guadagno, and Viko were at the house inside their compound. Elio was a mechanic, Rosa a midwife, Guadagno a nurse, and Viko a lab technician.

At the first sound of machine gun fire, closer than it had ever been in Beledweyne, Antonio and Carlo rushed to the compound. The seven foreigners gathered in the kitchen and watched through a window while heavily armed young men climbed over the wall and ran toward the house. They burst through the front door and the Italians put their hands over their heads in a gesture of surrender. The Somalis fired aimlessly into the kitchen. Antonio felt bullets zipping throughout the room. The smell of gunpowder filled his nostrils. Behind them, tomatoes exploded, splattering the walls with red juice and pulp.

The rebels ushered the hostages outside and forced them to kneel. Some of the rebels held grenades and pretended to pull out the pins. Others pointed their Kalashnikovs at the hostages' foreheads and mimed pulling the trigger. They raided the house and stole everything from Antonio's eyeglasses and Carlo's watch to all the food supplies, car parts, and personal documents. A few men grabbed Rosa and brought her into a room in the house, where they raped her. No one knew why they spared Annalena. No one wanted to talk about Rosa and what was happening to her while they sat helpless outside.

"We thought we were going to die," Carlo said. "In fact, we knew it."

The guards hired to protect the Italians ran away. Carlo said no one blamed them; he would have run away too. They didn't have sophisticated weapons and at least one was shot and killed as he tried to escape. Shaatos, who had followed Annalena to Jalalaqsi, raced to the compound when he heard she had been taken hostage but stopped before he came into sight of the attackers. He could do nothing and watched from a distance.

"I am a man of peace," Shaatos told me. "I never owned a gun. I didn't want the Italians to be harmed but what could I do?"

The hostages could see the body of the fallen guard. They tried not to think, not about the body, not about Rosa, not about what might happen in the next few minutes. Antonio cried a bit. Carlo was terrified.

"Only Annalena was calm," Carlo said.

There was so much confusion, for a few minutes Carlo contemplated making a run for freedom. He guessed the average age of the rebels to be fourteen years old and figured he could outrun them. But where could they go? All around Jalalaqsi was desert, no water, nowhere to hide. They had no car, no radio, and no money. And then he looked at the hand grenades and the rifles and stayed put.

For two hours they sat in the sun. Then the rebels loaded the Italians' generator into the back of a truck and ordered the hostages to climb into two separate trucks.

Annalena, Carlo, Elio, and Rosa sat in one truck, Antonio, Guadagno, and Viko in the other. Carlo was surprised to see a Japanese man in the truck already, but suddenly the rebels released him.

"Why did they let that man go?" he whispered to Annalena.

"He is not important," she said.

Carlo laughed. "Even while I was almost too scared to think, Annalena was calmly making jokes."

The hostages sat in the back seat of the Toyota crew cab, with two men in front and two in back, all heavily armed.

"We are taking you to Ethiopia," the driver said. "To Ferfer. No problems."

"Somalis are inclined to say 'no problems,'" Carlo told me, "but to us, there was a big problem. We were terrified." What would happen at Ferfer?

The trucks drove for hours, straight into the desert. For a while, Carlo said, it felt almost like a picnic. The hostages could close their eyes and imagine they were going to explore the desert, if they could forget about the guns, the robbery, the rape, the body back at the compound. Darkness fell and still the convoy drove on.

Suddenly a burst of gunfire came from one side and the truck carrying Carlo and Annalena swerved. In the darkness and urgency, the convoy divided, and the hostages were separated. The picnic mirage vanished.

They drove all night and in the morning stopped in a village for breakfast. Before anyone had a chance to eat, another truck approached around the corner of a house, this one with a machine gun welded onto the back. No one wore uniforms and the rebels thought the approaching men were on their side. The men in the approaching vehicle were government soldiers and thought the rebels were on *their* side. Each closed in on the other without shooting until they were close enough to look the other man in the eye.

Shooting erupted from all sides. Annalena, Carlo, Elio, and Rosa crouched down in the back seat. Bullets punctured the sides of the truck, one grazed Rosa's side. Elio was shot in the leg. All around them, rebels collapsed into the dirt. By the time the shooting stopped, every single one of their captors was dead but all four Italians were alive. They peered out the windows and waved their hands to show that they were unarmed. They tried to climb out of the vehicle, but Elio couldn't stand. Now that the adrenaline rush was over, agony surged through his body.

The government soldiers at first didn't realize they were looking at hostages. They thought the Italians could be spies or mercenaries and cocked their rifles, ready to shoot at the first command.

Annalena raised her head and one of the soldiers shouted, "Don't shoot!" He recognized her; she had cured one of his relatives of tuberculosis. "They are the Italian Medical Team."

That is one version of the rescue. Another is that a soldier recognized Elio as the mechanic of the IMT. They had once fought over the price of a jug of gasoline. Elio was tough, known for punching people when he lost his temper, or kicking them, as some remembered him doing recently to this soldier. Based on the number of TB patients Annalena had and the number of times Elio had beaten up people for trying to cheat him at his garage, it is possible both versions are accurate. In either case, the soldiers didn't shoot.

Now the four Italians were relatively safe, but they were still in a region surrounded by rebels, and Elio was bleeding profusely and in excruciating pain. The most comfortable place for him to ride was in the bed of the government truck, on a makeshift mattress alongside guns, ammunition, and bombs.

As they drove, the column came under occasional rebel attack and stopped to shoot back. Rosa, injured and traumatized, stayed in the truck, but at each stop Carlo and Annalena sought shelter outside and dragged Elio out, on the mattress. Every movement caused him to curse and shriek in pain. Annalena prayed out loud, over Elio's swearing, "God, forgive him, he doesn't know what he is saying."

Maybe she was sincere in her prayers, or maybe she just wanted to keep their spirits up and make people laugh. Carlo didn't mind either way. After doing this several times, Carlo and Annalena were exhausted and Elio nearly unconscious. They hadn't eaten or had anything to drink in two days.

"We weren't hungry," Carlo said. "Not at all. But thirsty. So thirsty."

They decided to stop dragging Elio out of the truck; it was too much for all of them. Under yet another barrage of bullets, Carlo and Annalena lay in the dirt beside the truck.

"Maybe I am going to meet my Lord," Annalena said.

Carlo was not happy about that prospect. "I am not inclined to meet him," he said.

"Oh, no problem," Annalena said, "You will see, I will introduce you."

Carlo laughed as he recalled this conversation; he repeated it several times, laughing harder with each rendition. "I had to tell her, please stop, or I really will kill you. I threatened her, and she laughed. Even Elio told her to shut up, to go meet her Lord alone. It was just to break the tension. I was really afraid, but she was calm the whole time." The thought of death didn't bother her.

"Maybe I will die from a stupid bullet," she said. "I will meet my Lord."

Again, Carlo wanted to punch her. Elio was in pain, Rosa violated, their coworkers probably murdered, death near, and Annalena said she would die from a stupid bullet nonchalantly as if they really were on a picnic.

The soldiers brought the Italians back to Jalalaqsi, where they dropped them off at a government building to rest. The well in the compound was filled with fetid water, but the Italians gulped it down anyway. They couldn't stay here. Rebels were scattered throughout the area and they needed to get to Mogadishu quickly or Elio would lose either his leg or his life.

Already Carlo could see the beginning of gangrene setting in. The bullet had pierced Elio's upper leg and he had a compound fracture of the tibia.

How were they going to get to Mogadishu?

Antonio, Viko, and Guadagno were not dead. After the first ambush, when the vehicles swerved and lost each other in the darkness, the driver of their truck stopped, climbed out, and grabbed his gun.

"Get out," he shouted at Antonio, the hostage closest to the door. Antonio obeyed, and the others followed. He felt certain they were about to die.

"Go. Walk. Go."

It was dark, and Antonio could barely see without his glasses. The rebels had stolen their shoes and shirts. Thorns, snakes, hyenas, and scorpions filled the desert.

"Go," the Somali repeated.

"They are going to kill us," Antonio said. "Run!" He hoped that if they ran in three different directions and were shot at in the dark, they would have a good chance of survival. All of them seemed to have the same thought and when Antonio said "run" again, they scattered.

"Probably the rebels were laughing at us," Antonio said, "because nobody was shooting. They just left."

There they were, three men stripped to the waist and barefoot in the desert at night. They moved away from the road, hid behind small bushes, and curled up side by side, partly out of fear and partly against the cold. At sunrise, they started walking in the direction of Jalalaqsi.

After walking for hours, they came to a village. There were no cars here, only an ancient, rundown bus. Antonio offered to rent it.

"It is very old," the owner said. "I don't think it is able to move; forget about going all the way to Mogadishu. It will break. It will cost you a lot of money."

"I am going to buy it," Antonio said. He was exhausted, desperate.

"You don't have any money," the owner said.

"I will drive it straight to the Italian embassy and they will pay you anything." Antonio didn't care what the man charged. He didn't care if the embassy paid or not. He just wanted to get in the bus and out of the desert.

Once the villagers realized the men truly intended to drive to Mogadishu and that the ride would be free, paid for by the Italian embassy, at least fifty more people clambered on after them. Antonio drove straight to the embassy.

There, instead of finding relief, Antonio found himself in another fight. Diplomatic staff were angry he had agreed to purchase the bus, and they blamed him and the rest of the Italian Medical Team for remaining too long in Jalalaqsi. He was furious. These were the same people who had ordered them to stay after all the other foreigners evacuated, who had sent them to Jalalaqsi, who were supposed to rescue them. He argued with them for hours to find a plane willing to search for the others.

A massive Italian ship, the Galibaldi, sat in the Gulf of Aden, with plenty of helicopters onboard. Antonio begged for one of these. But Italian Ambassador Mario Sica refused. Finally, someone suggested hiring a private pilot. They found a young man willing to fly anywhere, even, the pilot said, "to find the devil."

The next morning, now the third day since they had been taken, the pilot contacted the soldiers with Annalena and the others. They arranged a pick-up location. When the pilot landed, no one was there. He radioed Mogadishu and said he would leave.

"No," Antonio said. "If you leave them now, Elio will die. They are on the way."

"I'm not afraid," the pilot said, "but Somalis are coming out of everywhere, toward the plane. You said to meet them here, there is nobody. I'm leaving."

"No. Stay there," Antonio said.

A few minutes later, Elio, Annalena, Carlo, and Rosa arrived. They boarded the plane. Immediately upon landing in Mogadishu, Carlo, Elio, and Annalena went to the SOS Kinderdorf hospital. There were no other qualified surgeons, so Carlo, shaking from dehydration, hunger, and exhaustion, performed the first of many surgeries to save Elio's life and leg, this one to remove the bullet. Annalena stayed beside Carlo the entire time. Immediately after surgery, the two men flew to Italy. Antonio, Viko, Rosa, Guadagno, and Miriam left shortly after. Annalena stayed behind. She met them at the airport the day they left, with gifts. She gave Antonio a piece of wood one meter long, with the first chapter of the Koran scrawled on it in swooping Arabic. It hangs on the wall in his home.

Over orecchiette, sun-dried tomatoes, mozzarella drenched in olive oil, and wine in Pordenone, Italy, Antonio recounted stories of his time with Annalena. Sometimes his eyes filled with tears, sometimes his wife Monica reached across the table to hold his hand, and sometimes he stopped talking and gazed over my head, lost in a memory.

"What did you discover about Annalena that surprised you?" Monica asked me. "What are you learning?"

I was quiet for a moment. "When I started to read about Annalena's time in Wajir," I said, "I felt like a failure. I also came to Africa, to the same region, and thought I would do some good, help some people. But it turns out, I'm a mess. I'm selfish and lazy. I could never have lived the way she did. I read these letters and think she really was a saint, more than human, not of this earth." I was surprised to feel tears prick at my eyelashes. Monica nodded, her own eyes bright.

"But I don't think she would want me to think that way. I don't think she would have judged me. She would push me, challenge me. She makes me want to live better, to love people better."

Antonio and Monica exchanged a silent glance. Antonio left the table and returned with a blanket in his arms. Red, with shimmering blue and green leaves embroidered along the edges. He held it out to me, over the flickering lights of two candles. I sat, frozen.

"Take it," he said.

"That was hers?" I knew the answer. It was the blanket she had slept on in Beledweyne, instead of a bed or a mattress.

"He wants you to have it," Monica said.

"I can't take it." Now I was crying in earnest.

"She would want you to have it." Antonio's voice caught. "She would."

I touched the cloth and then gathered the blanket up in my arms. The transaction felt sacred. I thought Annalena had changed my life after a man pointed a gun at her at the TB hospital in Borama. That's true, she did. But now, as I learned more about this woman who tried to make others laugh while being held hostage, who made grown men cry as they recalled her decades later, who lived with such passion that her presence could still be felt in a piece of cloth, I realized she was changing me much more profoundly. Her impact was not just about where I lived. It was about how I would live.

12

Mogadishu

WAR WASHED OVER SOMALIA like a tsunami. Both the Italian government and what remained of the Somali government refused to grant Annalena's request to return to Beledweyne. From Mogadishu, she stayed in touch with coworkers, nurses, and some of her five hundred TB patients. In October, she sent one million shillings for them to buy food. Most of the local supplies had been consumed or disappeared into guarded storehouses to be sold at exorbitant prices. Millet, rice, and sugar sold "for their weight in gold."[1] Food aid intended for Beledweyne, even a convoy of eleven trucks escorted by airplanes, was commandeered by rebels and never reached the town.

On December 30, 1990, militants entered Mogadishu and the civil war broke out in earnest. That day, Bishop Giorgio gave the last Mass in Mogadishu to a somber group of Catholics. The sound of gunfire outside peppered the service.

The next Mass was canceled, but by then most of the foreigners had fled anyway. Eventually, escaped prisoners would break into the cathedral and dig up the bones of Bishop Salvatore. They would pry the gold fillings from his teeth and toss aside his skull. The building was robbed of everything of value, down to the rebar and electrical outlets. Homeless people slept, cooked, and defecated inside the cathedral.

January 26, 1991, rebel forces led by General Mohamed Farah Aideed closed in around Villa Somalia and Siad Barre fled in an armored tank. His flight left a power vacuum Somalis rushed to fill. Mariam Arif Gassem wrote, "One of Siad Barre's worst legacies is power addiction."[2] Everyone, it seemed, wanted to be in charge.

Aideed considered himself the ruler of Somalia, as his forces had done the work of getting rid of Barre. But Ali Mahdi Mohamed also declared himself president. Both men were Hawiye, belonging to different subclans, and the subclans went to war, decimating the city. Warlords, militia, and *mooryan* (gangs of young armed men) took over, often fighting to gain control over a single block.

Looting was wild and indiscriminate. From the US embassy to the National Theater, every building in Mogadishu was cannibalized. Violence ruled the streets.

Murray Watson, a British aid worker, described the early days of 1991. "I've just been round the hospital which is receiving betweeen fifty and sixty wounded people a day. Doctors are carrying out ten or fifteen amputations every day. I've got blood on my feet. You cannot imagine the carnage. I took some photographs of bodies in the street just now. There aren't so many bodies because the dogs have eaten most of them. But there are still hands sticking up through the sand."[3]

Annalena saw the bodies in the streets too. She described a woman's body among the corpses. The woman wore a military uniform and a *garbarsar*, "the veil a symbol of femininity, dazzling, tied to life," now forgotten among the dead.[4]

Almost every morning when Annalena opened her front gate, she found a fresh body, dead by bullet, by starvation, by disease. She hired dozens of Somalis to work as gravediggers and sent them throughout the city to find the bodies of those who had died during the night, and to give them the dignity of a proper burial.

"Why did you stay?" I asked Claudio Croce, an employee of SOS Kinderdorf, who worked in Mogadishu during the war.

"I believed in the project," he said.

The same questions tumbled out during interviews, even though I am annoyed when people asked them of me, over and over. Weren't you afraid? Was it safe? Why did you stay?

The default expectation is fear and self-protectionism. Armed body guards, blast walls, barbed wire, armored tanks. This makes sense for military personnel. But for humanitarians? How can a person help the people without being among the people? Tossing food sacks from the back of a truck guarded by armed soldiers makes great television but doesn't solve the intractable problems at the root of hunger or unrest. It can even prolong conflict and leave vulnerable populations open to worse crises in the future.

The organizations that came to Mogadishu with recognizable names and massive budgets, such as the International Committee of the Red Cross, spent $50,000 a month on security at the port. Media organizations housed their staff in hotels and villas that cost over $20,000 a month. They hunkered down behind prisonlike security measures and only ventured out surrounded by guards, whom they paid several hundred dollars, basically bribing warlords not to kill them.[5] Thousands of starving Somalis set up camp inside the football stadium. Aid workers visited but some wouldn't even go inside, citing the danger to themselves.

Then why visit? Did they come just to observe? To satisfy their curiosity and write an interesting report? To advance their own careers and salaries? That's what Annalena suspected. She saw how their money – bribes paid at roadblocks, salaries to gunmen, exorbitant piles of cash paid for gas and food – propped up the very warlords who caused the displacement of the thousands inside the stadium. And then, with their caution, the aid workers observed.

That isn't exactly true. They won grants, spent money, wrote reports. They made plans. They liaised with governments. But it's also true that they didn't manage to change much. Scott Peterson writes in *Me Against My Brother*, "Professional do-gooders were routinely compromised by their own humane intentions. And Africa's warlords have taken full advantage. Civilians are the target of atrocities, and armed groups steal relief supplies, manipulate aid to further their war aims, and kill relief workers when they don't get their way."[6]

Annalena mostly worked at two hospitals in Mogadishu: Forlanini and SOS Kinderdorf. Forlanini housed tuberculosis and psychiatric patients. Prisoners broke out of jail during the war but patients with mental illness remained chained to beds, unable to escape the shower of bullets and grenades, unable to find food or water or to clean themselves. Annalena brought them food and water.

The SOS Kinderdorf Children's Village treated women, children, and the elderly. The Austrian aid organization partnered with three nuns. Sister Maria Antonia worked in the maternity ward. Sister Bernardina sewed green uniforms for the Somali surgeons. Sister Marzia was in charge of pediatrics, medicine, and food.

SOS provided housing, food, and medical care. Tuberculosis was never far from Annalena's mind, even during war. SOS seemed like a possible partner, if she could turn their attention from crisis intervention to disease and prevention.

Claudio Croce met Annalena in Mogadishu to discuss opening a tuberculosis project at SOS, free of charge, for mothers and children.

Annalena wanted to keep the tuberculosis patients separate from other areas of the hospital. She wanted to require people to stay twenty-four hours a day, for six months, which raised issues of food supplies, security, and accommodations. She insisted on a certain treatment method. She was uncompromising.

They couldn't reach an agreement.

"Annalena was a problem," Sister Marzia told me. We sat in an empty classroom at the Caritas school in Ali Sabieh, Djibouti. Our conversation was in Somali, our only common language. She, in her nun's habit, speaking Somali with a thick Italian accent; I, in my khaki trousers, speaking it with an American accent. We laughed at the strange scene we must have made.

"She worked alone. Annalena wanted people to work with her but her character was very strong. And her life . . . she was unique, set apart. Many people came and tried to work with her, but they left."

For a while, Annalena lived with the nuns at the SOS compound.

"I have a whole room," she wrote, "with a delicious bed, bedside table, wardrobe, coffee table, desk, chair, even a ceiling fan."[7] It was the most furniture she'd had in one room in years.

"But she didn't sleep on the bed," Marzia told me. "She said she didn't want one and slept on the floor."

Speculating on the reason the women had trouble working together, Claudio said, "I think the sisters viewed Annalena as a lay missionary who aligned herself with the name Catholic but who wasn't really embracing the sisters' way of carrying out their mission."

"Annalena gave the impression she was doing the best work and the others a bit less," Bishop Giorgio told me. "She said, 'I am working for Somalis, others for expatriates.' This was completely wrong. The priests and nuns were really committed to Somalis too, just in a less exclusive way." He thought there was also jealousy of her commitment and success.

"I thought, yes, there might be different approaches. Let people do what they can, how they think best. But it is like when you drive a car and there are different gears. If you are going in second, Annalena is going in fifth. Probably her character was excessive," Bishop Giorgio said. "I was surrounded by these strong women who could not work together."

Sister Marzia told me nothing extraordinary happened during her time in Mogadishu. Ten minutes after our interview, my voice recorder was turned off when her coworker said, "Did you tell Rachel about the missile that came through the front door?"

"What?" I said. "No, she didn't." Missiles through doorways didn't matter to Marzia.

Marzia laughed. "I stepped away from the door and just then, boom! Everything exploded."

"Were you afraid?" I asked. There was that question again.

Marzia looked at me with what I can only describe as compassionate pity. "I'm not afraid of anything," she said. "True, there was risk. But all these women and children would die if I left. My own life is good. But I am one person. They are so many. So, we stay. Annalena was that way, too. We are not more important than them and we believe in heaven."

Marzia knew the risks. She was kidnapped once and only released after dozens of Somali women surrounded the house where she was being held. They sat outside for three days without leaving. When Marzia was freed, they threw a party in her honor. One of the guests sat next to her on a couch. He held a mug of tea and congratulated her on her freedom. It was one of her kidnappers. She thanked him for coming.

Annalena knew the risks and would have agreed with Marzia, at least on this point: their lives were no more valuable than the people they served.

Once it became evident that Annalena wouldn't be able to do her TB control program at SOS, she planned her departure. "I will organize an independent program," she wrote. "With Mario Neri."[8]

Mario had left Somalia, he thought for good, on March 22, 1991. He had married and divorced a Somali woman. He had treated patients in Beledweyne, four years before Annalena moved there. He had lost his voice and never recovered it, back in 1983. He had contracted Hepatitis C and lost fifteen pounds in one week, but doctors weren't convinced the loss of his voice and the sickness were related. Some blamed trauma. Some blamed exhaustion.

"Maybe it is some kind of paralysis in my brain," Mario told me. He sounded like a smoker, like it hurt to talk, and I leaned in to catch his words. "One day I got up and felt something strange, like when a person has to speak in front of a lot of people. A lump in my throat." After that, his voice was gone.

He'd also lost all remnants of the Catholic faith of his childhood, though he admitted that while working alongside Annalena it was possible to think maybe God existed.

That March, Mario and his coworkers flew to Nairobi. The lack of security had impeded all of their attempts at establishing a sustainable aid program in Mogadishu. They were disappointed but forced to abandon Mogadishu to her fate.

Mario couldn't shake the troubling sense that he should go back. The group of Italian doctors and nurses had only been in Somalia for one month. They had achieved nothing. He said this to the others, and added, "I'm going back."

They stared at him in silence. No one disagreed or tried to talk him out of it. They were all shell-shocked; they had only left the carnage behind one day ago. They could almost still smell the blood, still hear the bullets.

Mario wrote about his Somalia days in a book, *Lorenzo*, composed of letters to his son. He said the others knew what it was that pulled him back, even while they successfully fought against the pull. "The risk, the unknown, the desire to at all costs do something, to feel useful and alive."

On March 26, while his colleagues resettled in Italy, Mario found an open seat on a Belgian military flight. He carried no money, no luggage. At the airport he was picked up by a car filled with armed men. They drove him to SOS Kinderdorf. Wind blew dust around the car and the city seemed smothered in gray. People moved like ghosts between demolished homes, chunks of bombed cinder block, and piles of stinking garbage. The occasional gunshot pierced the air.

"My God," Mario thought to himself, "what have I done?" He remembers running his hands through his hair; at that time it hung down his back in a long, black ponytail. "It seemed suicidal. But I felt I must express solidarity with Somalis, even if only with my presence." And, as he wrote, if he had not returned, he would never have met Annalena.

At SOS, Mario was the only pediatrician, probably the only one in the entire country. [9] The hospital lacked everything from fuel to medical equipment to food. "There is no anesthesia in the operating room," Mario wrote. "There is no hope."

Annalena liked Mario and described him as sweet, a long-haired man who loved children and practiced yoga. "He speaks frankly and honestly and seems to know his limits. A great gift."[10]

They talked of leaving SOS together. Annalena wanted freedom. For her, freedom was not an ideology. Many Catholics, especially in South America, advocated a liberation theology that combined political activism with service to the poor. Annalena never became involved in politics beyond pleading with Aideed and Ali Mahdi to stop killing their people. For her, freedom meant the freedom to love, and it meant the freedom to love the way she wanted to love.

During the civil war in Mogadishu, however, freedom from a protective organization or from armed guards also meant the freedom to be killed. AK-47s sold in the market for seventy dollars. For less than the price of a goat meat meal, men could buy two full clips of bullets.[11] Onions, tomatoes, watermelon, grapefruit, and cigarettes lined shelves alongside bazookas, machine guns, and hand grenades. Separating from SOS would expose Annalena and Mario to greater danger.

While the battle raged for Mogadishu, Barre mounted a counterattack in the hinterlands. Fighters from his subclan rampaged through the agricultural regions, destroying farms and looting stored grain and food supplies. What had once been known as Somalia's breadbasket turned into a wasteland. Food became a weapon. Particularly hard hit was Baidoa, an area that earned the nickname "The Triangle of Death."

One aid convoy by the International Committee of the Red Cross made the controversial decision to hire armed guards to protect their delivery of fifty trucks stacked with seeds, beans, and rice. Upon arrival at their destination, the eighty guards mutinied and halted the food distribution, demanding seven times the originally agreed-upon payment.

The United Nations would normally provide security to assist such distributions, but when it came to Somalia the UN was slow to recognize there was a problem at all. And so, people starved to death while stockpiled food donations rotted at the port and gunmen filled their own bellies and pocketbooks.

Finally, in August 1992, Western media "discovered" the famine in Somalia. It had already been killing for months and before it was over, one third of children under the age of five would be dead. Peterson cites what he calls "headlines algebra" for Western news organizations, "One dead American is equal to a handful of dead Europeans. Hundreds of Asians might die to 'rate' the same treatment. And, bottom of the list, shamefully, are the thousands of Africans who must die before their tragedy will measure up at all."[12] This was true of the famine in Somalia and it remains true in terms of diseases such as tuberculosis.

After our lunch in Vicenza, Italy, Mario wanted to show me a lake. The drive was longer than I expected. Then he veered off the paved road onto a narrow grassy lane that descended steeply. The further we drove into the forest, the narrower the road became. Soon trees brushed against both sides of the car and I wondered what would happen if we encountered another vehicle. The thought struck me that I didn't know Mario Neri very well and no one knew where I was. I had no friends in Italy to call. I was completely at this stranger's mercy. But I didn't feel afraid. The next night, I was scheduled to sleep at Antonio Gabrielli's house in Pordenone and the following day I would have a meeting in Cesenatico with yet another man I had never met before. But Annalena trusted these men. Annalena was my connection to them. If she trusted them and they loved her, which clearly they did, I would be safe.

The day was warm and by the time we walked the four miles around the lake, sweat seeped through both of our shirts. Mario talked about his Somali ex-wife, his current wife and their son, the time General Aideed had a cold and called Mario to his villa for a medical check-up. My questions about Annalena had taken Mario down a road of nostalgia.

"Those days were the top of my life, really," he said quietly and gazed out over the lake. "The top of my life."

In April 1991 Annalena wrote that the SOS hospital was so low on milk there was no hope of saving the malnourished children. "The house shakes from war. They continue to bomb. We are surrounded by heavy vehicles. If we live, I will serve to the last breath."

The next day Annalena continued the letter. "Forgive me if I can't tell you all I would have said if I was not under bullet fire and pain for all the dead, wounded, widows, children, broken families. . . . I can only hope that if I die, the seed will take root and give fruit."

Annalena rarely confessed weakness, physical or otherwise, and even when she alluded to it, she quickly changed the subject. One morning during the days of heavy fighting she wrote that she didn't have strength even to make coffee and suffered from violent headaches. She denied this had anything to do with trauma or exhaustion or an oncoming sickness but, "certainly because I am heartbroken that people are led to the slaughter."

"I can do very little for them," she said, "less than a drop in the ocean."

It was time for her and Mario to leave SOS and work on their own. Annalena had a plan to move to Merka and start a TB clinic there, where violence was less constant, but in the meantime she decided to concentrate on food delivery. *Mooryan*, or gangs, stole her car. Likely they transformed it into a "technical." Men sawed off the top of a truck or Land Cruiser and fitted 106mm anti-tank cannons, machine guns, or anti-aircraft weapons to the top. The weapons were adjusted horizontally for street battles.

Annalena hired women to cook food that Shaatos, who had moved with Annalena to Mogadishu from Beledweyne, purchased in the market. Pasta, tomatoes, fish – any food he could find. The women prepared it in massive pots set over charcoal or wooden logs. They stood while they stirred, using long wooden paddles. Smoke curled out from beneath the blackened pots. When the food was ready, Annalena loaded it onto a cart, rented a donkey, and walked the cart through Mogadishu from her compound to the Forlanini Hospital.

Getting to Forlanini was dangerous. Danger, Mario told me, was in the air they breathed. The houses they passed were like skeletons with hollowed-out eyes, staring, staring. Annalena walked close to the donkey for some protection from bullets and bombs. "I walk the streets filled with rubble and the wounded, defying death rather than abandoning my people," she said. "As if the war did not exist."

In contrast, she described the International Committee of the Red Cross, Doctors Without Borders, and UNICEF moving about Mogadishu with machine guns and canons hoisted on top of their Land Rovers, just like the warlords' technicals, surrounded by armed guards.

Annalena sensed her presence bothered these organizations. "I'm an eyesore to those who came here for $10,000 a month without being experts in any sense," she wrote to her mother. "I am an absolute inconvenience: esteemed, respected, covered in praise by Somalis, Italians, foreigners. But I'm bothering so many who count that I must get out of Mogadishu soon."[13]

Annalena was not only critical of the aid organizations, but also of Christians. She loved the people working with her: Mario, Shaatos, Antoinette, who came later, and other Italian and Somali volunteers. But "the people with me should be the religious people, those who believe in Jesus. They never come." She wanted Bishop Giorgio and others to join her in facing the dangers and work of feeding crowds of hungry children and mothers no longer capable of smiles.

"We are the only ones who risk our lives to serve the poorest. Others stay for their salary and others for the dream that they will one day convert these Muslims to Christianity. But no one with true interest in their joy, their fullness, their health, their serenity." She watched outsiders come from Nairobi for a few hours a month and hide behind bodyguards, calling themselves humanitarians. In contrast, she believed that "at times like this, it is natural to give your life, unnatural not to."

The violence and the anarchic nature of it increased until the only rule of law in Mogadishu was a rifle. One day while the women prepared sauce to carry to Forlanini, two bullets pierced the wall of the compound and punctured the pot. Sauce poured out into the fire and the women who had been stirring it ran away, terrified and screaming, "Annalena! Annalena!"

Annalena was inside her office, typing reports. The bullets left two holes the size of grapes in the pot. She didn't stop her work, but her intention to leave deepened. "I must abandon this monstrous capital," she wrote, "where to survive you have to steal or beg, even though there are ten planeload of khat a day in the market." Khat, a leaf that is chewed, is the Somali drug of choice.

Stray bullets weren't the only danger for Annalena in Mogadishu. Though she kept her faith to herself, Somalis knew she was a Christian and the city was becoming increasingly fundamentalist, influenced by Salafi Muslims from Saudi Arabia.

In 1991, Salafis showered Mogadishu with leaflets. The leaflets explained that white people, all of them Christians, had a mark tattooed on their buttocks as a sign of their pact with Satan.

Salafis brought more than this rumor to Somalia. They convinced local leaders to implement Islamic law – an eye for an eye, a tooth for a tooth – in the hopes that such extreme responses to killing would deter violence on all sides.

Annalena wrote, "Soon the city will be filled with people with no hands, no feet, no eyes." The violence was too widespread, too complicated, too constant, for any kind of law, even sharia.

In her own desperate attempt to end the fighting, Annalena pitched a meeting with General Aideed and Ali Mahdi. They knew about her work and respected her neutrality but would not listen to her pleas.

Antoinette was with Annalena during her failed visit to General Aideed.

Antoinette, now ninety years old, lived alone in an apartment building near central Forlí, Italy.

"I don't know if she will talk with you," Maria Teresa warned as she walked inside with me. "She said she might, but she could always change her mind. She is an interesting lady. She loved Annalena."

A petite, frail-looking woman answered the door and I could tell the frailty was a mirage. She stared, her lips tight and her eyes piercing. Her chin was slightly elevated, and the upper half of her body barely moved as she walked us into the living room. The immobility was due to Horton's disease and a painful stiffening of her neck. She refused pain medications because she feared they would addle her brain.

In 1991, Antoinette faced a shattering family crisis, which she didn't share. She opened her mouth, hesitated, then said, "Part of this story is only mine."

Later, Maria Teresa told me simply that Antoinette fled cruel family problems and ran to Annalena, where, even in Mogadishu, she found the tenderness she needed.

"I have a bad character," Antoinette said. "My parents, my teachers, they all said this. I'm not humble. I don't care. You don't want me? I'm a bad character? You can leave me. But there was a wonderful feeling between Annalena and me. She took me as I was, without trying to change me."

Antoinette shocked her family when she left for Somalia. She had never flown before, spoke only Italian, had no experience in foreign countries, and brought no practical skills or medical training. She didn't go with the goal of saving people or even serving people. She needed to escape her own broken life. Antoinette became one of the Italian adventurers dodging bullets beside donkey carts.

"Do you have any kind of faith?" I asked. Antoinette told me she had grown up Catholic but abandoned the church.

"I don't know what faith is," she said. "Annalena had faith, but her faith was love. I can't say what her faith was. I can say Annalena was love and if love is faith, Annalena had a mountain."

Antoinette recalled Annalena's visit to General Aideed.

Aideed agreed to meet Annalena and sent military men to pick her up. Antoinette was allowed to accompany her to his home but not inside.

"Annalena told me Aideed was very kind, he listened to her." But the meeting changed nothing.

A few days later, Antoinette and Annalena were home alone. A gun battle erupted in the center of town, so they didn't go outside. The sound of gunfire and roaring car engines came closer, and suddenly armed soldiers burst into the house. They shouted and waved their weapons, and stole everything of value.

"I was stuck to Annalena like glue, like gum," Antoinette said. "I didn't leave her side and her only thought was to protect me, to defend me from the soldiers. I was hanging on to her and she was afraid someone would hit me."

Maria Teresa interrupted Antoinette. "This gives testimony to the power of the lack of fear. Annalena told me many times that she never showed fear and she believed that was why she was still alive."

I tried to imagine if I would be the clinging, cowering Antoinette or the courageous Annalena. I've been called brave for choosing to raise my children in Somaliland and Djibouti, but I've never faced this kind of violence. The few times guns or bombs threatened my family, we packed our bags. My life here has been work and school and grocery shopping and holidays and volleyball games with friends. There is nothing uniquely brave about living in Africa.

Annalena and Antoinette were thrown into a car. Antoinette asked Annalena, "Are they going to kill us?"

"We will kill you," one of the men said to Annalena.

"You will do it," she responded, "Allah knows." She then turned to Antoinette and hugged her.

"Yes, they will kill us. But they will do it quickly."

The car drove all the way out of Mogadishu.

Suddenly, the car changed direction and brought the prisoners to the Doctors Without Borders compound. The kidnappers forced the Italians from the car – Antoinette remembered the men laughing dramatically – and then drove away in a cloud of dust.

"Why don't they kill us?" Antoinette asked Annalena.

"I don't know," Annalena said, "but I think those people were the same men who brought us to Aideed's place."

"Maybe," Antoinette speculated in her living room with Maria Teresa and me, "maybe Aideed, who honored Annalena, changed their plan."

Annalena wrote a letter about the incident and said, "I saw uncertainty in the eyes of those who plundered the house. With one hand stealing but with the other hand moving away those who would harm us."

From the Doctors Without Borders compound, the women were taken to the airport and put on a flight to Nairobi.

"We landed with nothing at all," Antoinette said, "except the clothes we were wearing."

"Don't worry," Annalena said. "We will go to Joe Morrissey's house." Later, at Joe's house, a package arrived. Inside they found piles of underwear for a plus-size woman.

"And we were both so skinny," Antoinette said. They laughed and laughed. "Instead of being desperate because we had nothing except this large underwear, we laughed. This is so typical. We were in a tragic moment, but we were happy to be together."

Annalena stayed in Nairobi, making plans to return to Somalia. Antoinette flew to Italy, but she wouldn't stay long. Within a year, Annalena moved south to Merka, Somalia, and Antoinette joined her.

13

Merka

MERKA WAS THE SITE of one of medicine's greatest
triumphs, though barely. Here, doctors accomplished what
Annalena could only dream of. Doctors and scientists have
only rid the world of one infection: smallpox. Had they failed
in Merka, Somalia, the result would have been global failure.

In 1977 Ali Maow Maalin worked as a cook at a hospital in
Merka. On October 12, a car carrying two patients, a six-year-
old girl and a two-year-old boy, both infected with smallpox,
stopped to ask for directions to an isolated medical encamp-
ment. Ali got into the car to provide directions and rode with
the children for less than a mile. The girl died three days later.

Ali came down with a fever on October 22 and left work
early. His friends and family thought he had malaria and
admitted him to the Merka hospital, where he had contact
with dozens of other patients as well as medical staff and
visitors. Four days later, Ali developed a rash. The doctor
diagnosed chicken pox. As a child, Ali had been afraid of
needles and was never vaccinated, and though he personally
suspected smallpox, he said nothing. He didn't want to be
forced into an isolation camp, like the one where the young
girl had died.

By October 30, Ali could no longer hide his illness and a fellow nurse reported it to the regional health superintendent, who informed the Smallpox Eradication Program. Immediate quarantine went into effect. A policeman and a soldier were on duty at all times until Ali was discharged. Officials identified 161 people who had likely come into direct contact with Ali. Each one had to show their vaccination scar and papers or be vaccinated again. All eight hundred occupants of the houses around Ali's were vaccinated, and officials closed the hospital. Police established checkpoints and anyone leaving or entering Merka had to either prove prior vaccination or be revaccinated.

Ali recovered, and no one else became infected. Smallpox was defeated.

Ali subsequently devoted his life to eradicating polio and educating people on the importance of vaccinations. He died of malaria in 2013.

While on the surface Ali's story looks like a victory because it ends with the eradication of smallpox, it is a tale of mistakes, luck, and problematic assumptions. Why was Ali allowed to get into the vehicle with the sick patients? Why had his lack of vaccination never been discovered? People assumed he, a cook at a hospital, had his vaccinations. They assumed a mere one-mile drive wouldn't be long enough for germs to transfer. And the story ends with his death from a curable disease, malaria. Because malaria doesn't affect the wealthy, little progress has been made on this deadly pestilence.

These same assumptions contributed to Ebola appearing in the United States in 2014. And they are the same assumptions made about tuberculosis, coupled with Western disinterest, because TB and Ebola aren't "Western" diseases.

Tuberculosis has not yet been attacked with an effort as unified as the one that eradicated smallpox, and it continues to infect millions of people every year. In 2012 the first two new drugs since the 1940s were developed for clinical use. There is still no effective vaccine. It can cost more than $200,000 in the United States to cure a case of multi-drug-resistant TB (MDR-TB).[1] Even in Africa, costs are prohibitive, ranging from $2,000 in Ethiopia to $20,000 in South Africa. Treatment can take two years or longer, and the patient may end up with permanent damage to the lungs, liver, kidneys, and hearing. A patient can infect dozens of people before his or her cure or death. This is not a disease to be ignored.

Journalists called Annalena the Mother Teresa of Somalia, but Somalis never called her that. They called her *hooyo*, mother. She wasn't a saint to them; she wasn't otherworldly or religious. She wasn't there to help them die. She was flesh and blood, not a religious symbol or icon but a woman with whom they had a relationship. She was there to help them live.

Helping Somalis live had never been more challenging than during Annalena's years in southern Somalia. The Wagalla Massacre was horrific, but it ended, and people could rebuild their lives. Somalia remained in violent chaos: an entire generation raised with bodies in the streets, no schools, shattered families, and weapons in the hands of children.

When Annalena moved to Merka, the city was relatively calm. Anything was calm compared to Mogadishu. She said Merka had the most beautiful coastline in the world. "Clear water, untouched beaches, white sand, red dunes, the blue-green ocean. The people are industrious and love peace. Merka is white under the moon while the muezzin calls and roosters assert their supremacy."[2] Within months, that untouched beach would be the graveyard of hundreds, mound after mound marring the view.

Annalena met with some of the men presumably in charge, Omar and Osman Sheikh, to explain her goal of opening a tuberculosis clinic.

"What weapons don't do," she said, "Tuberculosis will do. If Somalis don't kill themselves, TB will do it for them."[3]

It took three days to convince them that she didn't have religious motives. They talked about a coming holy war and told her that if she expected them to visit her clinic, she should cover her hair.

"I will not cover my hair," Annalena said. "You can just stay home."

Annalena wrote to Mario, "We need a doctor. If you want to come, it would be very nice for us." He came. Like Annalena, he had no organization, no salary. Antoinette returned. Shaatos moved south.

The middle of a civil war was a risky time to begin a tuberculosis control project. "Who can guarantee we can carry out our program and complete the treatment cycle?" Annalena wrote. "No one. It is a bold choice, to put hundreds on therapy."[4]

International relief organizations decided not to treat tuberculosis during the Somali conflict, though even before the war began treatment had been minimal, so this wasn't much of a change. The official stance on treating TB during war was that it was better not to start anyone on a therapy than to risk interruption.

Treating infectious diseases during what are called "complex emergencies" can do more harm than good. The UN defines a complex emergency as "a humanitarian crisis in a country, region, or society where there is total or considerable breakdown of authority resulting from internal or external conflict and which requires an international response that goes beyond the mandate or capacity of any single agency and/or the ongoing UN country program."[5] These crises mean staff, medicine, and equipment can't be guaranteed. Infrastructure is destroyed, hospitals have no electricity, trained personnel flee, sanitation is atrocious, and follow-up impossible. Treating tuberculosis in Somalia, many believed, would only contribute to multi-drug resistance.

Relief organizations talked about TB prevention or a vaccination campaign, even though the BCG vaccine had proven ineffective in stopping epidemic outbreaks. But neither of these projects was implemented and Somalis were dying. Annalena went against the conventional wisdom.

Her rented compound sat two hundred yards from the ocean and could be reached through narrow alleyways. Inside a wall, cement houses surrounded an open courtyard. There was no barbed wire or glass on top of the wall to deter thieves. "If they want to come in, they will be coming anyway," Mario said. "At that time thieves only wanted food or medicine. They weren't after foreigners."

Annalena also rented the houses on either side of the compound to house sick patients and to use as a school. The courtyard became an open-air ward. Annalena hired a local artist to paint whatever each patient wanted by their bed. Some chose the Somali flag; others chose wild animals, radios, or fruit. Patients were given spittoons and a nurse filled them with fresh sand each morning. One of the courtyards became the kitchen, another was for women who wove dried grasses into baskets to sell, or mats for patients when the beds were full.

Annalena and Mario each took one small room. She outfitted hers with a thin mattress, which she rolled up and placed in the corner during the day, unless someone else needed to borrow it for sleeping.

Annalena's office was on the second floor of the main TB compound, packed with boxes of medicine and canisters, a tower that nearly touched the ceiling. There were no screens on the windows to keep out mosquitoes and Annalena kept the shutters thrown open wide to give herself a view of the ocean. She had a wooden table with ledgers for recording expenses, income, and treatments. There was one manual typewriter and a stack of manila envelopes for carrying the piles of Somali shillings required to buy food or medicine.

In southern Somalia tuberculosis had as strong a stigma as it had in Wajir, but people were so hungry, traumatized, and afraid of more violent deaths that they couldn't summon the energy to mask their disease. Once news of Annalena's clinic got out, the sick poured in from the city and from rural areas. Most had tuberculosis, but others were simply starving to death.

Annalena sat behind her desk to greet new patients. She wore a stethoscope around her neck and worked out of a huge logbook in front of her. Her large glasses slipped in the heat to the tip of her nose as she interviewed patients about their symptoms, family situation, and background. She spent two to three hours on each intake interview. Once she knew names, she never forgot, even to the second and third family names. She took special delight in watching children's faces light up when she called them by name and in connecting family members with one another, based on their genealogies. This relational time was essential for the effectiveness of treating TB. The reason TB control programs failed, especially during complex emergencies, was because medical staff couldn't convince patients to complete treatment. They couldn't convince them because there was no relationship of trust, empathy, or true care.

"Somalis are smart," Marina Madeo, who replaced Mario after a few years, told me. "It's hard to gain their trust, but once you have it, they will never turn their back."

"How could she diagnose TB?" I asked Mario. They had no lab equipment.

"It is like a person with AIDS," he said. "When you see someone with TB, you just know. They are very thin, with a certain expression on their face. You don't need a lab." Eyes bulged, cheeks sank in, chests looked concave. They were weak, coughing, had no appetite.

Weight loss was the most obvious sign of TB. But, as journalist David Brown pointed out, this can be confusing in a country with so many malnourished people. He wrote, "The ambiguity led to a diagnostic rule of thumb: if you feed someone and he doesn't gain weight, he has TB."[6]

"As a doctor," Marina said, "the experience is incredible. These children are brought from the bush in a state of stupor, and you start to feed them and break the balance, and either they will die very soon or they will recover. It is wonderful when they start to smile, because that means they will recover."

Annalena said it even more directly: if people were going to die, they would die in the first two days. After two weeks of treatment, almost no one died.

"Resurrect is the most appropriate word for TB patients," Mario said. "They now sing, play, dance, shout at the blue sky their desire to live. If I had left, perhaps many of them would now be buried beneath the white sand."[7]

What started as tuberculosis treatment for a few turned into a program for over a thousand TB patients housed in a hundred houses throughout Merka. Mario also ran a feeding program, with two thousand children.

"I can't sleep," Annalena wrote. "Tormented by starving children. They are too tired to even call me *galo*, infidel. They only say, 'I'm hungry.' I feel so inadequate."[8]

Children came to the center so emaciated they looked like old men, their skin stretched over their bones. Some were carried or pushed in wheelbarrows; others stumbled along on bare feet. When staff fed them, they bit into their own fingers as they brought the food to their mouths. But if they lacked the strength to feed themselves or ate too slowly, someone, sometimes their own mother, snatched the food from their plate either to eat or to feed to a more valued child. Survival of the strongest was the rule; the weak person was a burden.

When children arrived at the center, many of them collapsed in Annalena's or Mario's arms, desperate for an affection their parents could no longer give.

"Love?" Mario said. "Can you even use the word? Maybe, yes. I look at Annalena. She is a person who loves unconditionally, totally, unreservedly, a great love like the sea – clean, bright, clear. Nothing is expected except being able to demonstrate love. What luck to be here with her. To witness at the same time as tragedy, a boundless love."

Fifteen or more children died every day. Inside the compound, women sewed and cooked and nurses treated the sick, but outside, the war arrived in Merka. Bombs exploded and gunfire shattered the quiet every morning and afternoon.

I couldn't understand how Annalena stayed. Mario, Marina, and Shaatos also stayed, and gave me their reasons. But no one stayed as long as Annalena and each of them credited Annalena with giving them courage and endurance.

I found part of an explanation in a letter in which Annalena asked Marina to bring a guitar when she came. I think Annalena made a choice, a conscious decision, to focus on joy and hope. Had she focused on sickness and death, she would have despaired.

Often Somali women, the mothers of the dead children, seemed to turn cold. Some of them laughed when their children died. Others appeared unaffected by the deaths of their entire family. One woman lost three children in a car accident when a truck lost control in the market. Within days, she was back at work emptying bedpans of patients with diarrhea. She would talk only of Allah's will.

These seemingly passive reactions to death, reported by Westerners, turn Somali mothers into monsters. Nothing could be further from the truth. Loss after loss has pummeled these mothers. Their catatonic stares and arms frozen around lifeless infants show the depth of their grief. The brain and emotions have shut down in the face of unfathomable trauma. Immobility and the lack of wailing or tears don't make for compelling television. But how dare we who observe from a comfortable distance demand a woman reveal the intimacy of her devastation to strangers to prove its veracity?

One Western journalist wrote in the *Somali Journal*, "These traits [of apparent coldness] made it possible for Somalis to endure and seeing them makes a visitor's denial easier also. There is just enough strange about everything – the language, the weather, the politics – to keep a person like me from fully imagining the misery."

To focus on Somali mothers' lack of evident affection or grief gives Westerners a way out, a way to distance themselves from the horror of famine, war, and disease. If these women aren't visibly grieving, they must not love their children as much as we love ours. It isn't far from there to the conclusion that these atrocities aren't so awful and we can return to our regular television shows without guilt.

Annalena taped a list of the Wagalla dead to the wall of her Merka room and said they often came to her in her dreams, one by one, during the night. But in the morning, when she woke before sunrise and sipped a cup of *kawa*, Somali coffee, she would look out the three windows of her room that opened onto the sea and watch boats bob and sway in the silvery-gray water.

"The sky is clearing," she wrote. "A new day. God is not yet tired of men."

She met Mario and Shaatos in the TB clinic by six o'clock. Shaatos sometimes arrived shaken, or late, because he was forced to dodge bullets on the short walk from his home. Or he would be unable to leave on time because of a battle too close for safety. They spent the next three hours treating TB patients and preparing food.

Mario focused on the children. Many suffered from kwashiorkor – severe protein malnutrition – or needed feeding tubes, too dehydrated to drink. Worms plagued many of them, some as long as spaghetti noodles. They burst from children's throats, almost suffocating the kids, or emerged from their ears and eyes. Some children needed surgery, but without reliable electricity Mario struggled in the dimly lit spaces even to find veins for inserting a needle.

"Many times I wondered if I would get out alive," Mario said. "I wondered if what we did made sense. Maybe it would be better to leave without interfering, without presuming to change history, leaving this country to find its own way, even if through a bloody path."

Later in the morning, Annalena would go to the market to bargain for food. She refused to pay bribes and insisted on fair prices, but still spent more than eight hundred dollars a day on fish, spaghetti, biscuits, milk, tomatoes, and rice. She hired Somali women, most of them patients in the clinic, to cook the food; Shaatos helped distribute it. Patients who were strong enough to walk came to the pots with tin cans sawed in half for carrying their food. The "rich" among them used plastic bags, somehow able to find fresh ones every couple of days. Annalena hand-delivered food to those too weak to leave their mats.

"She bent over like this to feed hundreds," Shaatos told me. He stood and bent over from the waist with his legs held straight, like a Somali woman, and demonstrated dropping a biscuit into an imaginary person's mouth. "I asked myself, 'Is she not human like me?' It would be lunchtime and she would still be working. I would leave, eat a nice lunch, and rest a bit, my back totally aching. I would sleep thirty minutes, come back, and still she would be working. At night she would go home and eat a little tomato, a small salad, then start typing."

Annalena had back problems like Shaatos, but she didn't speak of them out loud.

Feeding and checking on patients continued until eight o'clock in the evening or until the cauldron-like pots were emptied of the last grains of rice or lentils. Only then did Annalena go home.

Some nights, shooting distracted Annalena from writing reports and letters. "Such a waste of ammunition," she said. Other nights, she admitted to exhaustion but still had work to do: washing clothes, preparing her small dinner, paying staff. She hired masons, painters, and carpenters to restore damaged houses and hospitals, even while bombs destroyed the city. Each person's salary was a way for her to fight back against the encroaching darkness of war.

Food quickly became a powerful and controversial player in Somalia's conflict. Feeding centers like Annalena's attracted people to the city and to camps where they often died of dysentery or measles, which they wouldn't have contracted had they stayed in the bush. While farmers and herders were away from home, their houses, farms, and animals were destroyed or looted. The very existence of feeding centers begs the question: If there is enough food in these camps, is there really a food shortage?

In Merka, there wasn't a food shortage. Annalena found all the food she needed for more than two thousand people every day. But she had to fight for it, she had to risk her life for it, and she had to pay for it.

Every financial exchange needed to be done in cash and the only way for Annalena to get cash was to have someone physically carry it to her. Bruno and Joe Morrissey arranged a system with an Alitalia pilot, Paulo Zambianchi, who lived in Nairobi. Bruno sent money to Joe from Italy, Joe brought it to Paulo. Paulo lined his pockets with dollars and stuffed money into old, used envelopes intermingled with letters destined for Somalia. Paulo flew into Merka and carried the envelopes directly to Annalena's table, where she dispensed medicine.

When Paulo was unable to arrange a flight, he sent the money with Somalis, again mixed with letters and regular post, and often on a khat plane, the only daily flights guaranteed to arrive in Somalia on schedule. These envelopes could contain over $30,000 total and militiamen brought them to Annalena's clinic.

"These militiamen loved me," Annalena said, "because I gave their people life. They brought the mail and would shout, 'Annalena, your mother wrote to you again!' They told me I was so lucky because people from all over the world wrote to me." They never suspected they were transporting thousands of dollars, and Annalena claimed she never lost a single dollar.

There was money and there was food in Merka. So why were children dying every day of starvation? Why did their bellies bulge like water balloons and their skin sag and their mothers stare listlessly while their infants wailed?

Large aid organizations move slowly and have global policies that can't be adjusted, at least not in a timely manner, to account for local circumstances. Mario talked about the policy of "no control" over food distribution, which led to the inevitability of it being looted.

Arranging security details didn't ensure proper distribution of the food either. Money paid for security went directly into the hands of the people causing the conflict or doing the looting.

President George H. W. Bush said that seven thousand tons of food aid was "literally bursting out of a warehouse on a dock in Mogadishu while Somalis starve less than a kilometer away because relief workers cannot run the gauntlet of armed gangs roaming the city." [9]

Annalena didn't ask why other countries, aid workers, and even other militaries should be brought in and put at risk to feed a nation. She saw people who needed to be fed, the innocent and the children, and she fed them. Not by bribery, not by military force, not by displays of power.

She believed in small actions, minor miracles. "I had no power. I was mother, sister, integral to their lives," she said. "I was not an NGO," a non-governmental organization, "with a satellite phone, waving my flag. Those people are in danger of doing good without love." [10] She begged NGOs not to flaunt their work, to do good covertly. But they couldn't. They needed the money provided by massive publicity campaigns. They advertised their presence, handed out branded t-shirts, and soon became targets of violence and were so restricted in their movements that their work made little impact.

"People [at NGOs] are fighting for prestigious positions," Annalena wrote. "It is a horrible abomination. The luxury of their homes and offices amidst people who are hungry." All while failing to feed the people they were in Somalia to feed. "It is pathetic. Aid planes come and only drop a few boxes, but they always have enough room for photographers and journalists."

Somalia was so dangerous that at Christmas in 1992, President Bush had announced a US military intervention: "Let me be very clear. Our mission is humanitarian, but we will not tolerate armed gangs ripping off their own people, condemning them to death by starvation. . . ."

Elsewhere, Bush reportedly said, "If the US can make a difference in saving lives, we should do it. No one should have to starve at Christmastime. We come to your country for one reason only, to enable the starving to be fed."[11]

If no one should starve at Christmastime, not even in a Muslim country where no one celebrated Christmas, was it okay for them to starve at other times of year? And how did President Bush imagine military personnel would ensure the delivery of the food? Did he have a plan to end the conflict, so food aid would no longer be needed, or did he expect to be in Somalia interminably?

Mario and Annalena discussed food and security. "Peace is not at the door with guns," Mario said. Annalena agreed. She believed peace would not come until Somalia was emptied of weapons.

"But what should be done?" Annalena asked. "Abandon the country to her fate? To the slaughterhouse, which will occur slowly, a trickle of untold innocent suffering? It is easy from the outside to say people should be left to kill, free to choose their life as they die. We have to live with the people to realize there is no way out."[12]

When do outsiders step in, and how? And when do they stand idly by? To most, it seemed the options were military intervention or impotency. Annalena forged a third way.

The military handbook American soldiers eventually received for Operation Restore Hope said, "Somalis admire military strength and power."[13] Annalena and her motley crew lived in the opposite way. Through humility and sacrifice, they saved lives and brought productive work, meaning, dignity, and education.

I don't think Annalena would have stayed in Somalia with only a feeding center. She needed to be involved with tuberculosis; that's why she had left Mogadishu. She knew the issues of food aid and the complicated relationship between donations and warlords, the way aid perpetuated conflict. She also knew Somalis had enough food to feed themselves, that when the shooting stopped, they would figure out a way to survive and rebuild. She wasn't there to do what Somalis could do, and should do, for themselves. What Annalena brought was a unique skill set and access to medication without which people with tuberculosis would die and would infect thousands on their way to the grave.

To ensure that she wouldn't contribute to MDR-TB, Annalena had to guarantee a steady supply of pills, either delivered in planes or through the port. Since the 1970s, Merka's port had been barely operational, abandoned by Siad Barre in favor of the larger, closer Mogadishu port. But the war rendered the port in the capital practically impossible to use.

In January 1992 Annalena convinced elders to reopen the Merka port as a channel of wealth. They could receive and sell goods; it would increase communication with the outside world; food and medicine could arrive. She wrote to her mother, "Rejoice because it was your daughter who worked hard to reactivate it."

Because of the danger of getting medicine via the Mogadishu port, Annalena had refused to put children on a TB regimen, but now she felt confident they could treat more, so she increased the numbers of pediatric patients, much to Mario's relief.

Some doctors came. And left. "Where are the people?" Annalena would ask Shaatos. "We have plenty of resources. It is the people who are not here. We need people – people with good hearts and determination."

During a rare interview she gave with David Brown of the *Washington Post*, Annalena said she required people stay at least six months. David came to Somalia as a medical reporter. She told him someone with no experience in the Third World would require one to two years before they would be useful. Brown wrote, "Like every demand she makes, it is exacting. But, she asks, what is it I am asking for? Time. Only time. It is the one corner you can't cut if you want to cure TB."[14]

Annalena wanted people to come for four years. A month, one year – such short commitments led to work that didn't last and didn't make an impact.

But how long could she herself stay, as the violence increased around her?

14

Complex Emergencies

ANNALENA STILL DIDN'T want publicity and David Brown's articles about her are some of the few in which she allowed someone in close. But she didn't want him to photograph her. "Who I am does not matter," she said. "If you do something for others, nobody should know about it. I believe this absolutely." After his articles were published, she started receiving cash donations, some as small as five or ten dollars, some even from Americans in prison. But overall, Annalena didn't have positive experiences with journalists. One, Greg Myre, called her an angel among Somalis and the Mother Teresa of Somalia, the earliest instance of this comparison that I could find in print, "pulling off small miracles every day." [1] She told him not to write about her.

Annalena didn't want to be a saint or Mother Teresa or an angel or a white savior. She didn't want praise or attention. She wanted to be left alone to do her work. The journalist can't grasp her love for the people or her willingness to sacrifice, so he frames the picture in the only way that makes sense to him. The local woman, the mother with a dead child in her arms, turns into a monster, or a ghost, and the foreigner becomes a hero. There is little context, little background, no interaction with the mother who has perhaps buried seven children and a husband, whose grief renders her immobile.

"We care for these children," Dr. Marina Madeo said, "for months, nursing them back from cholera or TB or starvation. And reporters come and want to know about the numbers. These children were not numbers to us. They were people."

When volunteers did come, if they made it past the first few weeks, the shock of war, the trauma of death, and the brusque reception from Annalena, they often stayed much longer than their initial commitment. Marina planned to stay for six months. Annalena barely glanced at her when she arrived. She stayed three years.

"Annalena is part of me," she said. "Her life was like the fruits of life and light passing from one person to another."

Fundamentalists trickled to Merka from Mogadishu and Annalena tried to avoid them. If they realized her potential, how she had hundreds if not thousands of supporters among moderate Somalis, the work would be at risk.

"They won't be happy for a Christian to have such popular esteem and gratitude," she wrote. The words indicated a striking shift toward religious violence targeting foreigners. "I have no illusions. If there is a 'holy war,' we are doomed. I'm not worried about martyrdom but about the practical impossibility of serving the poor."[2]

In May 1992 men shot at her house and someone delivered a handwritten note, "Annalena must die!"

"It would be laughable," Annalena said, "if it wasn't so exhausting."

Her patients made a public demonstration. They waved signs and blocked roads. "Our mother must not die," one of them said in a speech. "Her death would be equivalent to our death."

The warlords backed down, this time. But in June, gang members barged into the TB clinic and demanded Annalena pay "rent" for the right of a foreigner to work in Merka. She refused. They grabbed a few of the sick, patients too weak to resist, and threw them into the street. Annalena watched without raging or crying, which would only have escalated things, as they ransacked the compound, stealing medicine, food, and mattresses.

She bought back everything they stole, down to her Bible and one of her favorite books, the letters of Etty Hillesum.

"How many people do you think she cured?" I asked Bruno. People said hundreds, thousands. They said she gave millions of dollars over the years, hired hundreds of staff, saw hundreds of people educated. What were the numbers? I wanted to count them, to measure her success. NGOs always counted, even if the numbers in reports were far-fetched or reprints of other reports' hypothetical numbers. At one point, a UN report printed in the *Washington Post* said up to 4.5 million Somalis were facing starvation. At the same time, some estimates placed the entire population of Somalia at 4.5 million. NGOs count their effectiveness by how many meals they've served, how many children they've fed, while the qualitative question they should be asking goes unanswered: How does this aid increase overall and long-term food security?

Bruno didn't want to talk about numbers. "The heart of the message is not how many she cured." He wouldn't attempt an estimate; no one in Italy would. But Somalis lined up to tell me how she changed their lives. They provided the qualitative answer.

"I would have grown up illiterate but now I am director of a high school."

"I would have finished school at third grade. Now I am an investigator in the national police."

Lawyers, politicians, the first deaf person to be headmaster of a hearing school, pilots, businesspeople. They all credited Annalena not only with their career success but with the quality of their character.

"She made me who I am today," Elmi said. He planned to retire from politics within six months of our conversation. He wanted to return to Wajir and work among the poor. And he wanted to develop history lessons that included Annalena and her role in the region. The lessons would teach religion, science, and international affairs.

Numbers do not matter, Bruno said. "The heart is to serve humanity and above all the most unfortunate, the most unloved. This is the heart of Christianity. It is not prayer. It is service."

"She saw a wounded man and didn't see Christ," Roberto said. "We never thought of heaven. Our heaven was earth and our Eucharist was the poor. We could stay without Eucharist, without Mass, without prayer. Our faith was the poor. It was a call from humanity."

"The poor are waiting for us," Annalena said in one of her few public statements. "The ways of service are infinite and left to the imagination. Let us not wait to be instructed in how to serve. We invent and we live the new heavens and the new earth each day of our lives. . . . If we don't love, God remains without an epiphany. We are the visible sign of his presence and we make him alive in this infernal world where it seems that he is not. We make him alive each time we stop next to a wounded person."

Her motivation flowed out of the conviction that in the actual act of service she, in partnership with this needy person, revealed God and his love to a broken world. Through living in poverty, she would enter authentic and mutual relationship with the poor and through those relationships, she would experience Jesus. This turned the ideas of service, love, and mission inside out. People of faith talk about the "call" of God. In almost supernatural ways, they feel God's voice direct them to move to a certain place, to engage with a certain group of people, to spread their faith. As they follow this call, they discover the poor. Annalena saw poor people, lived in solidarity with them, and there, she discovered faith.

"We have no power," Annalena wrote. "It seems that I will end as a religious martyr. Maria Teresa would say I am to crown one of my all-time aspirations. I could die in a trivial incident at any time – a stray bullet, a projectile – or I could survive to old age. Only God knows."[3] Just a few months later, she wrote that she was too powerful. Not because of money but because of her reputation and the numbers of people in her care: one thousand sick, one hundred and twenty employees, now spending one thousand dollars daily at just one of her many care sites.

Everything had a price, and everything could be bought. When it became clear in Merka that at Annalena's clinic people had food, work, and education, some of the tuberculosis patients sold infected sputum to healthy people desperate for a safe bed.

After Annalena bought back the items the gangs stole in June, she was robbed again in July. At night, two thieves broke into her house. The thieves were known criminals who had murdered several people. They tied Annalena to a chair with her hands behind her back. One of them held a knife to her throat and demanded money.

"Kill me," Annalena said. "God exists."

"Where is the money?" the man said.

"God exists." Thousands of dollars for staff salaries were in a cardboard box beneath a shawl, a few inches from Annalena's chair.

When the man asked again and grew nervous and agitated, Annalena told him she had a small amount of cash at Mario's house. The thieves grabbed a few items from her room, mostly books, and ran. As soon as they left, Annalena worked her way out of the ties on her arms and rushed to the window.

"Thief!" she shouted. "Thief!"

"Thankfully they just ran away," Mario said. "Instead of coming to my house. Annalena found great comedy in that."

The first words Annalena wrote after the attack were, "We are still alive." The man who tied her to the chair would be hired a few months later by the Red Crescent to receive shipments at the port.

"It seems sadistic," Mario wrote. "Someone is laughing at us. I have so much need of serenity, peace, silence, and space. Instead, I am destroyed by these children for whom my science can do nothing."

Sometimes Mario shouted that if God existed he clearly had no care for humans. Or that God didn't exist at all.

"What kind of Father is this?" he said. "Where is he?"

Annalena had no assurances apart from what she called her own "rocky faith" – the only time I know of that Annalena ever wrote about a personal faith crisis. "Where are the honest people? The trustworthy? Sincere? Respectful? Merciful? Where are the peacemakers? In the abyss of evil, those who have faith are at risk of losing it."[4]

Mario found small comforts to give him endurance, usually in the evenings over dinner. After dark and after every patient's needs had been seen to, Annalena and Mario ate together and debriefed about the day. Annalena had taken two boys orphaned by tuberculosis into her care, Saad and Abikar. Their rambunctious play lightened what was, generally, a weighty darkness. Throughout the evening, Annalena would scoop up one or the other, hug them tightly, and kiss their cheeks.

"Children don't understand the violence," Annalena said. "They hear the guns, pause, and then go back to playing. It is a mercy. And, babies keep being born. Some are even little fatties, as if they were born in paradise instead of hell."

Mario prepared coffee for Annalena and mixed it with sugar, one of her few indulgences. Mario's weakness was for chocolate, and Annalena brought him chocolate bars whenever she traveled to Nairobi.

They made a concerted effort to eat in a dignified manner. A cloth covered the table and ironed napkins were placed beside the plates. The glasses were turned upside down until the meal began. Annalena complained that eating her meals hot made her spend too much time on them.

Even though her back ached and she took several pills a day, albuterol and anti-inflammatories, she was tempted to rush through meals to get to her typing work: letters, reports, budgets, and patient files. She suffered from the climate as well, with a near-constant pain across her chest and difficulty breathing. She battled migraines. She suspected one particularly painful headache was aggravated by the tension of the twenty-fifth anniversary of her arrival in Africa. Another headache she attributed to both air conditioning and an endless speech she had to sit through, given by an Italian diplomat. She had malaria several times.

"We all had malaria," Mario said. "But she didn't stop for a little fever."

Over dinner they debated the merits of their work, the nature of God, the value of staying versus leaving. Mario said they faced a hopeless abyss.

"I see hatred and wickedness, without remedy." He felt bewildered and embittered, so immersed in hell that no other reality could be true.

While he questioned the existence of God and the goodness of humanity, Annalena questioned herself.

"I have learned," she said, "or rather understood deep inside myself, that when something is not going right – incomprehension, arguments, injustices, unfriendliness, persecutions, divisions – surely the fault is on my side. I can be sure I have made a mistake somewhere. At the feet of God, it is easy to find one's fault; it doesn't take long. It makes us suffer but not too much because it is so beautiful to recognize one's guilt and to fight for forgiveness, so that wrong ways can be reformed. My duty in this world is to be life-giving. Every error comes from my inability to love. How hard is my heart!"

I asked Bishop Giorgio about this focus on her own faults when surrounded by such evil. He had just told me of his arrival in Mogadishu the day after Bishop Salvatore's murder.

"How can you keep loving Somalis?" I asked. "How could she?"

"You say loving people," Bishop Giorgio said, "but this is the wrong question. It is not loving the people. It is loving Jesus. He makes it possible to love even our enemies."

I asked Maria Teresa too. Quietly, she said, "Jesus Christ. This is the real Jesus Christ. To love the unlovable. It is impossible."

At least she acknowledged the impossibility of Annalena's love.

"Many times, we finish," Mario told me, referring to himself and Annalena and anyone working in desperate places, "and we think: What have I done? Was it a good thing or not? Was it better for me to stay or not? But when you are there, you feel healthy. You see the immediate result. In that moment, you feel helpful. If you save the life of someone, it is a life. That's something. But in the long run, you say, what happens to the people I saved? What future do they have? The Somali children, where are they now? What have they done? Maybe they are criminals. Maybe they died of other diseases. But is the solution to do nothing? It is to help, but in what way?"

Annalena left the philosophical questions to Mario. She knew they couldn't solve the world's problems and made the decision to love the person in front of her. "I learned to bend my head in front of the mystery of pain, suffering, and evil. I do not want to know why. I will not torment myself unnecessarily. There is no answer. It is the mystery hidden from the foundations of the earth."

Mario still hasn't stopped asking why, though he knows the answer will always elude him.

In October, Mario wrote, there was an attack. A confrontation between two rival groups started with shouting over food issues and clan identity. The clinic stood between the two. One side launched a grenade and it struck a truck. Three of the four men inside were killed instantly. The legs of the fourth man dangled out of one of the doors and the truck skidded backwards from the impact of the grenade, shredding the man's leg against the wall of the clinic compound. The truck burst into flames. In the fire, the machine gun attached to the top of the truck came to life on its own, spewing bullets in every direction. Mario called it deadly popcorn.

As night fell and the rivals couldn't tell each other apart, the fighting slowed.

"Where was Annalena?" I asked Shaatos.

"She was an iron lady," he said, "Iron. No fear. Bullets and warring factions and she is typing. Wow-wow-wow!" he mimicked the sound of gunfire. "Here is her coffee," he held out one hand with an imaginary mug in it. "She is drinking, the rest of us are hiding." He recounted their conversation.

"Annalena, don't you hear what is happening?"

"Yes," she said. "But what do we do, Shaatos? What do we do?"

"Aren't you afraid of what might happen?"

"But what can we do? I must work."

"Fine. You continue to work, and we will continue to hide."

Shaatos turned to me. "And that's what we did. I hid under the desk with the others. Annalena drank her coffee and kept typing."

She was practical, as well as fearless, about the possibility of death. The money in the letters via Joe Morrissey had to be hidden somewhere. There were no banking options. She tied the cash, as much as $10,000, in a plastic bag and strapped it to her body. One day she brought Shaatos into her room and showed him where she kept the bag.

"You know there are bullets everywhere," she said. "If a bullet hits me, you remove this money. If I die, you tell the people to put my body in a private room, then you come and lock the door and take this money out, then open the door."

Shaatos prayed he would never have to do that, never have to see Annalena's dead body.

Both Saad and Abikar were dead by the time I talked with Mario.

"Why did she choose those two boys?" I asked.

He shrugged. "Life and death are a mystery." He told me about a girl he cared for. Maybe the only way to understand why Annalena did what she did, why Mario made his choices, was through stories.

Early in the morning on May 18, 1992, the guard at the clinic brought a seven-year-old girl to Mario. She was sick with active, late-stage tuberculosis, naked, emaciated, and unable to stand. She struggled to breathe and looked at Mario with wide eyes. She couldn't speak, and he never learned her name.

Mario had treated hundreds of children and could recognize when they needed more than TB medications, when they needed care and affection, without which the medicine would be worthless. He saw that in her eyes and decided to bring her to his room. He clothed her and carried her feverish body to his room, feeling her heart gallop against his chest. He knew she was near the end of life and the lack of oxygen would torture her for hours. He hoped to provide a bit of comfort and parental care before she died. She refused to swallow anything he offered.

She slept on the mattress and he slept on the cement floor, ready to wake at any hint of improvement or of suffering. During the third night, she moaned. Mario came close and she turned her head slowly, to look him in the eye. She took his hands and squeezed them, then she kissed them gently. He started to weep. He cried the rest of the night.

In the morning, Mario brought her to his surgery ward, so he could keep an eye on her. Some time that morning, she asked for spaghetti. He rushed to the kitchen to cook noodles and brought them to her. She nibbled slowly. A few hours later, she died. Her body was buried on the beach alongside hundreds of other children he had tried to save.

"I can't tell you a rational explanation for why I took this girl to my room," Mario said. "But in that moment, when she kissed my hand . . . maybe in that moment she felt someone with her and recognized she was not actually alone. In that way, maybe just for one minute, you show one person that you are there. Even if you can't save him or her, you are there. But to explain this," he started to cry while we talked, "why one and not another? It is difficult to say."

I had no response. Silence settled over us.

"I think that moment was the top of my life," Mario said. "I have never lived so intensely as in those moments when death was so close. You feel you are not divided as a person, you are one. The spirits come together. It goes beyond love. It is just one moment and then it is gone but in that moment, you feel something so strong, maybe you feel the divinity."

As much as Annalena avoided publicity, news about her leaked out. Other aid workers called her the last good Italian left in Somalia. Some said she "singlehandedly outstripped anything the UN achieved."[5] Others said she had time for everyone and was never distracted. "It is a very saintly characteristic," they said.[6]

Journalists, aid workers, and volunteers flocked to Annalena. Mario called their trek a pilgrimage. Annalena said they looked at her with a "veneration with which one looks at saints,"[7] and could barely tolerate their visits.

"Patients have the right to me," she said. "I can't spend time with guests. I understand they feel entitled to come and have my time, but they need to respect my needs. I'm not a monster who doesn't need anything, but if they respect me, they should please not come."

No one listened to her pleas to be left alone. Italy awarded her a medal of service and sent a warship to the Merka port for a ceremony. She tried to get out of attending, but the Italian ambassador and other officials waited, and she couldn't ignore them. A helicopter delivered her to the ship. After a series of speeches that she found interminable, she accepted the medal.

She didn't look at it, didn't care about its value. She sent it to her mother. "This Somalia is unbearable to me," she wrote to Maria Teresa.

Now, late in her life, Annalena said she realized that she never had to go to Africa at all. She could have loved the poor in Italy. But since she was already there, in the Horn of Africa among Somalis, she stayed. Had Annalena sought recognition or praise, she would have left Africa years ago.

For all her innovation in tuberculosis control, one of the most powerful humanitarian success stories on the continent, the medical community was slow to acknowledge her role in the development of DOTS. In 1993, she wrote, "After much slander and persecution, the manyatta policy is recognized as the only policy of effective protocol in the field of TB control for nomadic and semi-nomadic populations. They tell me I was a precursor, a voice in the desert. And I still am." Seventeen years after she developed the system, professionals in the TB world finally acknowledged that she had achieved her goal – the successful treatment of TB among nomads.

"Many do not respect me," she wrote, "because I am not a doctor. They demonstrate an insane jealousy of what I managed to do."

This, along with the war and disappointments with promised aid, contributed to a deepening exhaustion in Annalena. "Yes," she wrote to Joe Morrissey, "you read that right. I am exhausted."

The UN designated 1993 the "Year of Indigenous Peoples." Somalis called it *Dadka Cunkii*, the time of cannibalism.[8] And by early 1993, Mario had had enough.

"I take care of children condemned to die. I watch them slowly die of untold suffering. Not just physical suffering but suffering due to a lack of love, loneliness, hatred, the indifference of a world that refuses to see. Four hundred and fifty die in three months and that's only in Merka. A question plagues me: What right do I have to prolong the suffering of these children? What can the world offer them except war and pain? What about tomorrow? A month, a year from now? Will they have a dignified life?"[9]

He craved peace, silence, and space to run. He'd been doing yoga in his small room and ran in circles around a tiny carpet, but it wasn't enough. He struggled to broach the topic with Annalena. Part of his desire to leave was fear and, compared to her, he felt like a coward. By this time, Antoinette had returned to Somalia. Mario confided in her. The two practiced conversations, Antoinette playing the part of Annalena. When Mario felt sufficiently prepared, they went to Annalena together.

Mario started to talk but never got to the part about leaving. "He practiced it with me so many times," Antoinette said, "and at the time of saying it, he couldn't. And anyway, I had already told Annalena what he was going to say so she was laughing and laughing."

As part of a celebration to say goodbye, Annalena asked American soldiers to accompany them to a bay just outside of Merka, with some of the children he had treated. Finally, for one afternoon and under armed guard, Mario ran along the beach and up and down the sand dunes. One month later, in March, Mario boarded a C-130 with a group of Italian soldiers and left Somalia.

"The soldiers are silent with their thoughts," Mario wrote, "and I with mine. No, I'm not thinking. I do not know what to think. Suddenly, I feel drained."

Marina Madeo replaced Mario as the resident physician. She brought the guitar Annalena requested. Marina didn't play, but some of the patients did. Annalena sang along to the Somali songs while she and Marina wound their way through the crowded TB wards.

Annalena renovated space for fifteen classrooms, the only functional school in Merka during the war. She had nine hundred students in kindergarten through fifth grade.

"So," she wrote, "people are dying outside. And inside, children shout, 'kow, laba, sadex, afar, shan!'" One, two, three, four, five. "LIFE!"

In the fall of 1993, fundamentalists took over the dilapidated Merka government hospital and demanded all medicine and food pass through them.

Annalena received a letter from a group called the Somali Liberation Committee with three demands. One, she must hire three militiamen as guards and pay them comfortable salaries. Two, she must accept the guards chosen by the Somali Liberation Committee. Three, she had to prove there was a line item in her budget to account for the salaries of these guards. If these orders were not followed, Annalena was not welcome in Somalia.

Annalena responded with a letter of her own. One, Annalena does not worry about the risk to her life. Two, Annalena already hires the children of militiamen to work as guards, bricklayers, and electricians. She does not need to hire those chosen by someone else. Three, Annalena cares for the sick and oppressed and is not looting the country. She challenges anyone to speak out against her facts, even after her death, should she die. She concluded her letter with, "God is here. He knows."

Annalena could no longer guarantee medication and needed to stop TB treatment. "Because I can't bend to blackmail," she wrote, "I have decided to freeze the TB program, which requires commitment and longevity. Instead, I will prepare everything for the educational and social activities to continue in my absence." [10]

But she couldn't quit immediately and leave people in the middle of their treatment. To close the program without letting *mooryan* or warlords know and without promoting MDR-TB, Annalena stopped taking new patients. She would remain for six months, to train the staff and finish the current courses. She wouldn't leave until the last patient swallowed his last pill. Even in leaving, her love for the sick guided her decision.

Tensions rose. One afternoon while Marina was with the children and Annalena was in the outpatient clinic, a man walked straight up to Annalena and punched her in the face. The patients rallied to protect her. She continued to stand and stared at him, hard, in the eyes. He ran out of the clinic. A few weeks later a man struck her cheek with the butt of his gun, fracturing her left cheekbone. The injury left an indent and an ache for the rest of her life.

If it were only the violence against her, Annalena likely would have stayed until her death. Death threats came, handwritten and threatening to cut her body into pieces or to throw her to wild dogs. "My death, my illness, my pain is not different from the death, illness, and pain of those dying every day on the steps of my house." But the reality that she no longer had access to TB medications forced her departure.

She continued to trust and hope that all the evil she saw in Somalia would be exposed one day. "I have experienced that there is no evil action that does not come to light, no truth that is not revealed. The important thing is to fight as though the truth already existed, so that injustice does not weaken us, and evil does not triumph."

Talking about leaving was one thing, actually leaving was another. The *mooryan* expected Annalena to pay them, despite her letter of refusal. She came up with a plan, which all her staff approved. Shaatos had already left Merka, after receiving death threats because he belonged to the wrong clan. Caritas was ready to take over running the schools and feeding program. The TB medicine supply dwindled and then finished.

On August 9, 1994, Marina drove to the Merka airport to fly to Nairobi. Her term of service was finished. Annalena rode along in the car. Marina had her few belongings, Annalena wore a stethoscope around her neck. Marina climbed up the steps to board the plane. Annalena climbed after her, to say goodbye.

Suddenly, Annalena disappeared from the doorway, into the plane. The door shut, the plane rolled down the runway, and they were gone.

That night militia came to the clinic with guns and demanded to speak with Annalena.

"You want her?" one of the staff members said. "You'll have to go to Nairobi."

Maria Teresa came to Kenya to spend time with Annalena. She alone could convince Annalena to eat lunch: a few pieces of potatoes, some bread. Maria Teresa told Annalena to rest. Annalena wrote, "Strangely, Maria Teresa seems to believe I work too much, resulting in extreme fatigue of the rest of the people to keep up with me."

After resting in Nairobi and reconnecting with her friends and adopted family from Wajir, Annalena returned to Italy.

This time, she felt certain she would stay. She needed prayer, time in hermitages, and time with her books. She told Bishop Giorgio she had a double vocation – service to the poor and a hermitic life – and was constantly torn between the two. But were they really separate vocations, or was each a necessary part of the other? Maybe they couldn't be pursued equally at the same time, but without her hours or days or years of solitude, would her service have been so powerful? Without the stripping and exhaustion that came from serving in a world shattered by disease and violence, would she have plunged to such depths during her quiet moments with God? She once told an audience:

> In my life I have known many dangers. I have risked death many times. I have spent years in the middle of war. I have experienced – in the flesh of my people, those I loved, and in my own flesh – the evil of man, his perversity, cruelty, and wickedness. And I have come through it all with the unshakable conviction that only love matters. Even if God did not exist, only love would make sense. Only love frees people from all that holds them in slavery. Only love allows one to breathe, grow, flower. Only love makes us unafraid. It is for love that we risk our lives for our friends, that we believe everything, endure everything, and hope in everything. And so, our life becomes worth living, becomes beautiful, filled with grace, and a blessing.[11]

Annalena still didn't fit into life in Italy. Her nephew Andrea called her a foreigner. She brought only her two long dresses. Andrea said she slept little and always on the floor. He noticed the dent in her cheek and asked her about it. Her response was nonchalant, "Must have been a gun."[12]

Bruno took her to a restaurant to have a good meal. She ate only salad and a small ball of mozzarella.

"Look," Bruno said, "I took you here to eat good food."

"You don't understand," Annalena said. "I like this food."

"She didn't smile when she was in Forlí," Maria Teresa told me. "She was forced to stay in a culture she didn't like. Sometimes, when she was able to find a place to serve, I could make her laugh."

As soon as she could, Annalena fled Forlí for hermitages. She knew her family, especially her mother, were hurt by her long absences.

"If I say what I feel, I'd only hurt you," Annalena wrote to her mother. "You would feel judged and perhaps condemned by your choices." But then she said what she felt, anyway. "I can't live in your world. Everything seems so pointless, so unnecessary. The words, gestures, activities, things." She wrote to Bruno and Enza as well. "I am rich because you are rich, but I cannot stay in your house. It is too beautiful. The food is too much."

Her family and the diocese in Forlí pressured Annalena to speak at events. From her solitude, Annalena directed her mother on how to respond. "I will not talk in public. I want nothing more than hiding, silence, a chance to think and meditate and study. Advertising is not my way."

She didn't want to talk about the horrors she had seen, or about Somalia, or about international aid. "I now know what wins in the end is big business and that aid to the Third World is for enriching the giver. It makes him comfortable, revered, prestigious, powerful. Warlords want perpetual war – for power."

She feared people would use her stories to place her on a pedestal, to make her way of life seem too holy or too extreme for the average person.

She didn't have answers; she didn't ignore the grief. But she made a choice for faith, even if, in her words, it was a faith "shrouded in darkness."

Faith is mystery covered in that dark shroud, but love is active, evident, performed in the light. Many people in the West mix this up and think of love as an ineffable emotion and faith as a set of rigid dogmas and theologies to which one professes intellectual agreement. There was nothing mysterious about love for Annalena: it was service. It was physically caring for the needy. Faith, profound and intangible, wasn't where she looked for certainty.

Maria Teresa repeated lessons she and Annalena learned from Gandhi. "It isn't the multiplication of needs but the voluntary restriction of desire. Not only physical but intellectual restriction. And I, Maria Teresa, have taken the presumption to even add, spiritual. The restriction of spiritual needs to be able to serve mankind. If you don't limit your needs, you will never be able to serve."

The restriction of spiritual needs? How could someone so spiritual restrict spiritual needs? Only when she saw service as spiritual and rendered that service with no preconditions except love. Annalena left her prayers to sit at the side of dying TB patients. She took the Eucharist alone, without wine, in Muslim villages. She accepted insults, threats, and assaults without retaliation. All of this was love and service; all of it was faith.

Maria Teresa continued. "When you have reached deep inside you, in the cave of your heart, if you have reached the depth of your heart, your religion, the center, you'll find all the deepness of the other religions. The core. The others can dance, they can say Allah, Our Father, Buddha, but in the cave of your heart, you don't say a word. You are silent. And that silence can embrace all faiths. So whether someone says Allah or Buddha is not important. It isn't prayer, the holy books, the rituals. The only thing is this: the abandonment to the Most High, by any name you call it. Sometimes you may call it peace. God. You can call it anything. Catholics don't understand this. They feel I am forgetting Jesus."

She addressed my question before I asked it. What about Jesus?

"I think, really, Jesus is this. Take the pagan, the prostitute, even those who have no religion – he loved them. To love people is not religion. You forget about religion completely."

In other words, call God whatever you like. Live like Jesus. Love with absolute abandon.

In July 1994 an Italian doctor, Graziella Fumigalli, replaced Annalena in Merka. Annalena said Graziella was a champion. Smart, professionally prepared, with a great capacity for discernment. She was vigorous, fearless, and not willing to give in to blackmail.

At 6:50 a.m. on October 22, 1995, two Somalis entered the clinic and hunted down Graziella. They shot her three times in the face and she died instantly, with a pen in her hand and a stethoscope around her neck.

Annalena heard the news, wrote a condolence letter to Graziella's family, and made plans to return to Somalia.

SOMALILAND

1996–2003

15

Borama

WITHIN MONTHS OF GRAZIELLA'S MURDER, Annalena explored Sudan, Ethiopia, Kenya, and Somalia for a place where she could start another TB clinic. The search would bring her to a country that wasn't a country, a village that would love and despise her, and to a reckoning with her past choices.

In 1996, she visited Hargeisa, Somaliland. Somaliland was war-scarred but peaceful. In 1991, while southern Somalia collapsed into civil war and anarchy, Somaliland declared independence. Though unrecognized internationally, the region developed its own currency, flag, national anthem, and governing body. Slowly, the north edged away from the 1988 massacre and toward a more hopeful future.

Two Somali doctors were working in Hargeisa at the time, Drs. Qaws and Walhad. They faced several health crises in Borama and one of the biggest issues was tuberculosis.

"There is a lady I knew in the south," Qaws told Walhad. "We would be very lucky if she came to Somaliland. If she came here, she could cover all the problems."

Annalena and Shaatos toured the Ministry of Health and hospitals in Hargeisa. As Annalena approached one, a man sitting near the front steps suddenly stood up.

"Who is this person?" he said. "I know this person."

"Is that Dr. Qaws?" Annalena exclaimed, the happiness in her voice evident to Shaatos. "Imagine, Shaatos! This is Dr. Qaws. He was a medical officer in Bula Burte."

Dr. Qaws told Annalena about the tuberculosis crisis in Borama. All the same problems: a lack of supplies, poorly trained staff, patients who defaulted, the stigma around even saying "tuberculosis."

"Come, we will go to Borama and talk," Dr. Qaws said. He pointed at a Suzuki in front of the hospital. He was eager to go immediately, not wanting Annalena to slip away.

By November, Dr. Qaws achieved his goal. Annalena signed a contract with the WHO, the medical authorities of the Awdal region, and elders on behalf of the community. One official report of this agreement stated that Annalena was "nobody, just an individual supported for her projects morally and economically by friends and family."

Working out the agreement hadn't been easy and proved a harbinger of how Annalena would be welcomed in Borama. She continually emphasized that she was no one special, that she wasn't going to bring cars and money, that she was only an individual who came with experience working with tuberculosis. At first, people weren't happy.

The elders asked her to hire a plainclothes policeman to accompany her to and from the hospital. She said no. They asked her to cover her head with at least a *masar*, covering all her hair.

Maria Teresa and I went through photos I had accumulated. Some were from Bishop Giorgio, some from my own time in Somaliland, some copies of photos in newspaper articles. Few of them were labeled and I needed Maria Teresa to tell me what country Annalena was in, and who the people were around her.

The first photo I opened was of Annalena holding a small child. A flimsy purple scarf hung loosely over her hair and draped around her neck. Her graying hair was clearly visible. "This veil means she was in Borama," Maria Teresa said. "In Merka, Mogadishu, Wajir – no. She didn't cover her hair. But in Borama? The elders even wanted her to wear gloves and socks. She said no. She wanted to dress like a Somali but she didn't see the need to dress like a Muslim."

Postwar Somaliland was different from Wajir and Mogadishu. There was the semblance of peace, as there had been in Kenya. But there was also the recent memory of war, as there was in Mogadishu, and the destruction of infrastructure, so much so that when the first president, Abdirahman Ahmed Ali Tuur, sat in his office, he had no pens or paper. Control was paramount in the maintenance of peace and what felt like constraint to Annalena was an effort to protect her and, by extension, Somaliland.

While the government couldn't offer much help, wealthy residents in Borama provided Annalena with sheets, pillowcases, charcoal for cooking, free medication, and discounts at shops in town.

Professor Suleiman, one of the elders, said, "In Somaliland the government structure was just being started but was not strong enough to address security or lead the people. It was up to individuals and private institutions to fulfill that responsibility, to take up the slack where government is supposed to invest. It was against this backdrop that Annalena came and filled a gap – to help the poor, the sick, the disadvantaged."

There had been no TB control in over ten years in Somaliland. Annalena renovated the lab at the existing hospital and was given twenty beds for new intakes. On November 24, she began screening, and on December 15, she started treatment. That first day more than three hundred people showed up, but once they found out they were being treated for tuberculosis, only seventeen stayed.

Immediately, Annalena instituted what she called radical DOTS. "Not the fake type which is implemented in many countries, with the well-known consequence of being unable to stop TB."[1] She understood the "noble lie" of poorly managed DOTS programs – that they might look good in reports but actually be contributing to increased drug resistance. She also knew that the community of the manyatta system was vital to the success of treatment; people needed a larger context of care – not just medical but educational, vocational, and spiritual as well – in which they could thrive while they healed.

Annalena aimed to strengthen existing TB centers so that when expatriate staff would inevitably evacuate, local staff could remain committed to radical DOTS. She made all patients sign contracts stating that if they abandoned treatment a relative or some other proxy in town would be fined up to $150 and thrown into jail until they returned. Annalena probably wouldn't have implemented this on her own – she didn't like the idea of adding the stigma of jail to TB – but she couldn't allow people to default either. Early on, a few patients left mid-treatment. Annalena threatened to shut down new intakes. Borama officials arrested family members of the sick until they returned and rarely had to resort to jail or threats again.

Borama was hard. Her patients had been burned or doused in blood in the desperate search for a cure before giving Western medicine a chance. And she still couldn't say TB to them.

"*Shaqadaada ma lihi,*" people said. That's none of your business. They claimed a wind blew sickness onto them, or that their cough was due to falling out of bed, falling into a well, being kicked by a camel. Anything rather than face an infectious disease.

Her staff included four nurses, four assistants, a doctor, and a lab technician. The twenty beds quickly filled with people from town. As more and more nomads arrived, Annalena knew she needed to add an outdoor system of care, as in Wajir.

"In Somaliland, it was a tragedy," she said. "We had to use plastic tarps, not the beautiful curved wood, branches, or hand-woven mats Somalis used in Wajir." People shoved plastic bags into cracks to block out dust. They hammered tin cans flat to provide support. The huts looked like heaps of trash nailed together. Instead of handwoven mats, the ground was dirt and rock. Here, germs and bacteria lingered beneath the tarps, in dark, warm, moist conditions conducive to TB. The structures were also more permanent, with orange or green waterproof tarps provided by the UNHCR, instead of being built by the nomads themselves. Less ownership, less personal investment.

"The condition of the sick became terrible," Annalena said.

The condition of the hospital was also terrible. There was no generator and Borama electricity cut out between nine o'clock in the morning and six o'clock in the evening every day, all over town. Guaranteeing the medicine stayed at a constant temperature was one initial obstacle. It required a generator and an agreement with the electrical company. Quality x-rays were nearly impossible to obtain; they were foggy, blurred, and scratched. In the rare cases when Annalena questioned whether or not to treat for TB, she sent the scans to Italy. Biopsies also went to Italy. Sputum samples from possible MDR-TB cases went to Aga Khan Hospital in Nairobi. [2]

Annalena rented a house from Dr. Qaws and for a few months, before he married, Shaatos lived with her.

Their house, within walking distance of the hospital, was a simple cement block structure with a Western-style toilet, a sitting room, two bedrooms, and a small kitchen outside. Dr. Qaws hired a guard, Rashid, who came with his dog, Ruqiya.

At night, when Shaatos went to use the toilet, he would see lamplight coming from under Annalena's door, or smell incense burning. He knew she was either reading her Bible, praying, or typing.

"I learned to sleep, or not sleep, like Annalena," Shaatos said. "I became like Annalena." He stopped himself. "No, I can't say that. I can't say I became like her." He seemed embarrassed that the words had slipped out. I understood how he felt, from the time Maria Teresa had compared me to her. We could say we learned from her, were changed and inspired by her, but we couldn't say we were like her.

During the day, her yard converted into a kitchen. The hospital didn't have a kitchen facility, so Annalena hired four women to cook three meals a day at her house. Breakfast was tea and *lahooh*, a pancake-like sourdough bread. Lunch and dinner were sauce with rice or pasta, always with meat or beans. Daily, mounds of fresh baguettes heaped up in the yard. Annalena hired someone to clear stones and trash from the road between her house and the TB center so her employee, Daahir, could more easily deliver wheelbarrows or donkey carts full of food. Daahir ordered the firewood, pots, and pans, and Shaatos bought food supplies in the market. Shaatos also ran errands for Annalena. He tracked down defaulters in the bush, found new patients, managed the cooks, and purchased supplies such as blankets, mattresses, and pillows for the hospital.

Every patient had a wooden bedside table for a radio, medicine, papers, and their eating utensils, which they had to provide for themselves. "Often, cured people didn't want to leave," Shaatos said.

Days at the hospital started at 6:00 a.m. with a teaching time for nurses and lab technicians. Annalena conducted these lessons in Somali. While every non-Somali I talked to said she was fluent, Shaatos and other Somali staff said her language ability was merely passable. She had a thick Italian accent and couldn't make a "nice" sentence. But she was strong when making commands.

"She knew important words," Shaatos said. *"Adigu been ha sheegin."* Don't lie to me. *"Ilaah ka cabsado."* Fear God. And *"Run, miyaa? Haa."* Is that true? Yes. She also spoke in a southern dialect, intelligible to Somalilanders, but one more thing that set her apart.

In training, Annalena faced an uphill battle. Conservative women came swathed in cloth and wanted to be tested, or to receive shots, through their dresses. Doctors diagnosed patients without even taking off the sick person's jacket to listen to their chest. They prescribed the wrong treatments, mostly to suit the financial level of the patient. What people could afford to be sick with, the doctor told them they had.

When it was obvious a patient was about to die, nurses turned the bed to face Mecca and left the patient alone. Even before someone was near death, possibly to gain an open bed or because they didn't know what else to do, sometimes nurses left people facing Mecca.

It took time, as always, to convince the staff that total oversight of TB control was the only acceptable way. The morning trainings were required. By 7:30 a.m. staff began handing out medications. Annalena set up a table in a shaded part of the compound. Each patient had a folder with cards specifying their treatment regime and each brought a bottle of water to wash down the pills. The WHO provided the tuberculosis medications. Annalena bought aspirin and Tylenol from shops around Borama, and paid for medicine for people at the mental institution. Afternoons were spent on new intakes and visiting or attending classes. Annalena's voice could be heard over the walls of the hospital as she teased children at school or called out a greeting to a nurse.

"The problem," she said, "is not that the sick can't flourish but that they can't flourish if left alone."[3] To her brother she wrote, "The problem is the lack of genuine love. We do not love each other enough. We are not merciful enough to each other. We do not care enough for each other. We do not love our neighbor as ourselves."[4]

A well-known thief in Borama contracted tuberculosis. Forty years old, he had spent half his life in prison. People said the only thing he could do was steal and if he didn't steal, he would collapse. Annalena admitted him to the hospital.

"He was a real stray dog," she said, "full of lice and open sores. Everyone rejected him." Patients and nurses gossiped about him.

"He will plunder the pharmacy," one of the nurses told Annalena. Another claimed he would steal Annalena's purse or attack her house at night.

"Of course, I liked him immediately," Annalena said. "I called him Holy Moses."[5]

Every day Annalena asked Holy Moses where he had flown to in the middle of the night to do miracles. Many Somalis believed saints could fly, and her nickname bestowed an honor he had never experienced. He was shy but also proud, happy at her attention and a bit shocked that she would trust him when she had no good reason to.

"He didn't steal anything from us," she said.

About a month after his intake, he asked Annalena for a pen and paper and joined the Koranic school. When his treatment ended, he came with a larger batch of patients ready to be released. His clothes were spotless, his body washed and perfumed with soap. His skin peeled, though, from dermatitis, and he was embarrassed to greet Annalena.

"I promise you, I washed," he said, over and over. "These are blemishes. And I am very old . . . You must believe me, I washed and re-washed."

His body wasn't the only reason Annalena didn't step closer. "He didn't realize that it was also his breath!" she said later.

While TB remained Annalena's priority, the context of care for the entire person mattered more than any pill regimen. The deaf were nearly as ostracized in Borama as people with tuberculosis. Many people believed a person who couldn't hear also couldn't think, learn, or work.

"Our world is harsh," Annalena said, "a world of the strong with no room for the weak." She would always make room for the weak.

Annalena kept in touch with Mahamud, a young deaf man in Wajir. In 1997, he worked for a Kenyan coffee company and was engaged to get married. But when he found out his fiancée smoked and did drugs, he broke off the engagement. Heartbroken, Mahamud started walking north. He passed through Ethiopia, where he was arrested. Although he carried a valid Kenyan passport and had traveled to Italy and the United States, he had no visa for Ethiopia. Ethiopian police officers couldn't believe a deaf man could make it so far alone. Eventually, they released him, and he continued north until he reached Borama, and Annalena.

He thought maybe she would need a driver, but Annalena didn't have a car when he came. She wasn't sure what to do with Mahamud until she noticed that every night after working at the hospital, deaf people swarmed around him. He had learned sign language at Kerugoya and most of the deaf in Borama had never seen sign language before.

Amina Dahiye had already come to Borama when she heard Annalena was there. Annalena proposed Amina and Mahamud start a deaf school, the first of its kind in Somalia. They started with seven children gathered beneath a tree in 1997. By 1998, they had a building with four classrooms, a storage room, and toilets, all built by the UNHCR on land donated by the Borama community.

Seven students turned into twelve, and eventually fifty-two. Students came from all over. One day, while Annalena was doing outreach to find tuberculosis patients in the village of Aisha Adow, a little girl named Muna approached her. Annalena hugged her around the neck. The girl squeezed back.

"But who is this?" Annalena said. "I don't know this girl."

"Oh, she is deaf," someone from the village said.

"Then she is my girl," Annalena said. She spoke with Muna's parents and arranged for her father to work in a small store in exchange for transportation money to send Muna to Borama for school.

The school grew to include classrooms for hearing students as well, who were either disabled or belonged to outcast clans like the Yibir and the Midgan. Hearing students picked up sign language, to the dismay of their teachers, because they could cheat during tests without talking. As part of their education, students also learned embroidery, typing, and carpentry. They held weekly volleyball games and performed traditional dances. The school became so popular because of the quality of education and the community, even wealthy parents of healthy, majority-clan children requested spots for their children.

In 2002, Mahamud visited Eastleigh, a Somali section of Nairobi. He walked into the street and a *matatu*, a Kenyan minibus, honked but he didn't hear it. The matatu struck him and severely injured his knee. His mother came from Wajir to the public hospital and ordered the doctor to cut off the cast wrapped around his leg. She said there was "too much blood in him." She took him out of the hospital and brought him to a small clinic in Eastleigh where the doctor overdosed his anesthesia and Mahamud died.

Maria Teresa shook her head when she told me the story. So much death.

Zahara Abdillahi trained as a midwife in Somaliland.[6] She had been circumcised as a child and witnessed circumcised women give birth in extreme difficulty. Labor could last for days and stillbirths were common. In 1985, she worked in Yemen and attended a Yemeni woman's first birth.

"I took all my tools," Zahara said, meaning her knives and scissors for cutting through scar tissue. "Then I saw that a woman who had not been mutilated had no problem. She gave birth perfectly. I had never seen such a thing before."

Zahara returned to Somaliland where, in 2000, she met Annalena. Initially, Zahara worked at the hospital but Annalena proposed she start anti-mutilation campaigns.

UNICEF brought mosque leaders from around Somaliland to Hargeisa to discuss whether Islam sanctioned FGM. Sheikh Mohammed Sayeed Saweer from Borama was one of those leaders and he became the first religious leader to publicly speak against the practice. His wife had carried six full-term pregnancies, but each child was stillborn. He said it was because the birth canal was inelastic from scar tissue.

"Are you better than God that you tamper with his work?" he said. "Allah opened the mouth. Would you cut and stitch that too?"

Annalena hired Sheikh Saweer. She and hospital staff studied FGM for months. Then they invited women, women's political representatives, educators, elders, and religious leaders to a training.

"You will wonder why Borama TB Center is a promoter of anti-FGM activity," Annalena began. "Our center is not a typical center. We consider our patients as whole individuals and not simply as people suffering from a disease. Ours is a school of humanity.

"Our staff teach patients that health is not simply absence of disease but a state of complete, total, whole psychological, mental, and social welfare. Consider why we are here today. Female circumcision is also called female genital mutilation, because that expresses more realistically what happens. She is physically mutilated." Annalena compared FGM to war victims, people who lost arms and legs and suffered debilitating injuries for the rest of their lives.[7]

Someone interrupted her speech. "You can't speak in public about the vagina. This is a scandal and a disgrace."

Sheikh Saweer stood up with his Koran in hand. He affirmed there was nothing in Islam to condone FGM.

Annalena addressed an unspoken aspect of the complaint: her outsider status. "And why is this white woman talking to us about FGM? I am a European, but I have been directly involved with FGM. I adopted six Somali children in Wajir and brought them up in the Muslim faith. One of my daughters was brought to me by her grandmother – both parents died – when she was already circumcised. But the other two were babies when they were given to me by their families. And so, like all Somali mothers, I felt I had to circumcise my daughters."

Here it was, at last, a reckoning. How did she feel, publicly confessing this? When I read this quote, Annalena morphed into a much more complicated person than I originally expected to find. "I had to circumcise my daughters."

I had already uncovered minor character weaknesses, ways she offended people, physical pains she endured, and she had slowly become less saint-like and more human in my mind. But now, here was something she openly regretted. That, I deduced from the notes she made on the typed pages. She added two asterisks after saying she had to circumcise her daughters:

*because I could not render them different from the others.

*I feared that they might not be accepted in the society, unless they were circumcised.

She was defending herself. This revealed so much about Annalena: her growth, the depth of her identification with Somalis, her humanity, and her humility. This kind of cultural humility is what produces effective aid and development work. It is also what makes it so exceedingly rare.

Either because of a sincere delight in learning local customs, or as a reaction against outsiders' tendency to condemn or avoid customs that seemed strange, or likely a combination of both, Annalena plunged into Somali life. She adopted the living standard of people around her – their food, their love for the desert, their clothes and language. She hated the oppression of women when they weren't allowed access to education or were married off at young ages, but she strove to keep the children she brought into her home as authentically Somali as possible. From waking them at four in the morning to pray and eat breakfast during Ramadan, to reading portions of the Koran in her own prayer times, to circumcising the girls in her house, Annalena went along with the culture.

When is it appropriate for an outsider to speak up and challenge a local practice? I believe the answer is, when they have earned the right to do so. How does one earn that right? It is not through university degrees or official UN backing. It doesn't come through money or donations. It requires time and an openness to move beyond the surface. Many expatriates assume that if they learn some vocabulary, eat goat and rice, and adopt a semblance of local clothing, they have adapted. They're wrong. Gender norms, alliances, ideas of virtue, a hierarchy of character traits, value judgments – these things run much deeper. Until a person understands these, her commentary on a culture or practice will remain superficial and possibly offensive to the local population.

By this point, in Borama, Annalena called the fight to end FGM a "holy war." It was a war in which she had changed allegiances. Maybe the change came out of her experiences or her medical education. Maybe it came from knowing that she had earned a hearing among Somalis and could now more openly defy certain practices.

"We are in the year 2000 and our women are still suffering for a tradition that has no religious foundation," she said. She had lived among Somalis now for thirty years, and her use of the word "our" is telling. No outsider could get away with saying that. If a woman came from the UNHCR to fight FGM and tried to identify at this level with Somalis, she would be ignored at best. But Annalena had circumcised girls she considered her own daughters. Her willingness to be publicly honest about this set the standard for other mothers and midwives to come forward and change their minds too.

An elderly midwife stood up during the seminar. Kaladya Hadji had performed thousands of circumcisions and was known to be the "best circumciser in Borama." But being the best cutter didn't make her the most loved woman. She said young girls hated her; they prayed for death while Kaladya cut them. The memory of their cries made her feel guilty.

"I have known since Siad Barre started a campaign against FGM that this practice has no basis in my religion," she said. "And now I hear it from my own sheikh. I know I am a sinner. But, Annalena, if I stop, what will I do for my daily rice?"

"I will hire you," Annalena said.

"Then I declare in public that for the sake of Allah, I leave this."

She became a laundry supervisor at the hospital.[8]

Annalena, Sheikh Saweer, and Zahara opened an office. They created anti-mutilation videos, spoke on the radio, and held conferences. After one conference in Borama, the elders agreed to put up anti-FGM billboards at the entrance to the town.

Not everyone was supportive. People heckled the sheikh when he spoke. "What are you doing," they said, "taking money from infidels to come here and talk about our girls' vaginas? Have you nothing better to do?"

But twenty-eight women followed Kaladya's example. Annalena provided each with a $200 investment in the small business of her choice. One opened a restaurant, one began trading in used clothing, and another shipped vegetables from Ethiopia to sell in the market. Annalena also covered school fees for their children. At this point, she needed to raise $6,000 every month to cover all expenses and projects.

And then she added eye camps to her budget and schedule. Twice a year, she brought ophthalmologists to do surgeries on as many as eight hundred Somalilanders who had gone blind from cataracts. Plane tickets for the surgeons, housing, and supplies cost as much as $9,000. But she described the outcome as one of the most beautiful scenes a person could imagine: family members who hadn't seen the faces of their loved ones in over ten years, suddenly gifted with the miracle of sight, or children who had been blind since birth, now with their eyes open and healed.

Some of Annalena's projects were funded by the UNHCR or the WHO, but the Comitato in Italy continued to raise thousands of dollars every month.

Kitty McKinsey of the UNHCR, one of the people Annalena warmly but persistently badgered for more funds or staff or supplies, thought Annalena could have gotten more funding if she became part of an official NGO. Annalena told Kitty she didn't want to be required to fill out forms or do things the way other people wanted. Kitty saw her effectiveness and wanted to support it, but was constrained by rules and bureaucracy. "Everyone talks about empowering women," Kitty said. "Usually it is a vague concept with vague programs. But Annalena lived it."

Kitty acknowledged Annalena had unusual ways of talking about her work that didn't fit with traditional NGO language and often bordered on melodrama. She was "in love" with the sick, "called" to the poor. This was, of course, the language of faith, though not necessarily of a specific religion. When people asked how she as a Christian dialogued with Muslims, she laughed at the notion that this was complicated. "There is no dialogue, no seminar, no discussion. You live with them and everything is normal. Relationships are understandable. *Caadi*, as Somalis say."

The sick in Borama eventually accepted Annalena's treatment, and cures became commonplace. Each morning Annalena announced which patients tested negative. By now, though, at the end of their six months in the clinic, instead of being eager to leave, patients protested. They yelled that she didn't know what they had, that they were certainly still sick with TB.

"You have to treat me," one man said. "Why don't you treat me?"

"But you are negative," she said. "I can no longer give you the drugs."

"But Annalena, I know it. I am positive, I know."

"The first time you came here, you denied it and now you are fighting. Unbelievable!"

"Annalena, look, I'm coughing, look at my face. I lost a lot of weight. Can't you see? You are denying my disease."

When she managed to convince patients that they had "graduated from Annalena" as they called it, many of them returned several times in the following months. They felt like teachers and were proud to show off what they had learned about health, religion, and literacy. They told people to stop spitting, to wash their clothes and eating utensils, to avoid drinking dirty water, and to vaccinate their children.

One of her patients opened a *dukaan*, a kiosk, across the street from the hospital. Once healthy, he became wealthy and used his shop to give other people jobs. "I would not be alive if I had not gotten this treatment," he said.

"The breakthrough has finally come in full," Annalena declared.

But then, patients started dying – people who, on paper, shouldn't have died. Annalena began to suspect something more sinister was happening, and soon her fears were confirmed. Compounding the TB epidemic, AIDS had arrived in Borama.

16

The Nansen Award

ANNALENA MISSED THE COMMUNITY of like-hearted women she had had in Wajir. She missed the simplicity of the desert and the faith of nomadic Somalis who hadn't yet been influenced by fundamentalism. Maria Teresa said Wajir was the place where Annalena had been most happy, most satisfied. "She missed her desert Somalis, the ones from Wajir."

Bruno said Somalis in Borama, by comparison, performed the Islamic functions of prayer and Ramadan, but didn't seem as submitted. "They rebelled against tuberculosis treatments, against the heat; they were always fighting with each other," he said. It wasn't violent fighting like in Mogadishu, but the desperate fighting of a people coming out of war, now faced with limited resources. There was little margin. The fittest would survive and everyone struggled, clinging to the cusp of a prosperous future but dangling over a disastrous abyss. As Somaliland lurched forward into nationhood, individuals placed their own advancement above communal well-being, scrambling over one another to get ahead.

I asked Shaatos if Annalena was happy in Somaliland and he said she was, in a serious kind of way. Happy to do meaningful work. Others talked about her propensity for joking and making people laugh. But by the time she moved to Borama, she did less of this. She was tired.

"This is the growth of Annalena," Bruno told me. "She was young in Wajir, older in Borama. Her principal was the same – to live with the poor, to share. In Borama she started with her program written down and signed by the elders and the WHO; she wasn't just thrown in there like in Wajir. In Borama she could speak the language and push more." He paused. "She kind of grew up in Wajir but in Borama, she came in."

I suspect, too, that Annalena felt more pressure in Borama. She wasn't a beginner anymore, and there was no war to impede her. She wasn't young, no longer naïve. She had high expectations of herself and her coworkers. She had spent years developing her treatment and programs but struggled when people she hired took time to learn what she had learned. She thought of leaving.

"The last time I met her at the station in Forlí," Maria Teresa said, "she didn't even greet me. She said, 'Maria Teresa, I don't think God will keep me long in that place.'"

Joe Morrissey knew Annalena was lonely and visited almost every Christmas. But Borama wasn't a vacation for him. Annalena worked the whole time and he spent his days at the deaf school or doing tasks she assigned him. Christmas Day was no different. But after the students went home, Joe went to the hospital and waited for Annalena. They walked back to her house and, some years also joined by Bishop Giorgio, shared a clandestine Communion. She still had the bread of the Eucharist, the body of Christ, hidden in her room, as she had in Somalia. Usually the bishop brought wine. One year, Father Sandro came instead and he forgot the wine. Annalena said she would have enjoyed taking Communion anyway, but he refused. "Not everyone thinks like me," she wrote.

On Christmas Eve in 2000, Annalena called the Comitato. Her voice was dull and gave the group the idea she was repressing deep emotions. "Dozens of people die in the streets. We need expensive antibiotics to address the devastating impact of AIDS on the tuberculosis patients."[1]

Life as a lonely foreigner among the dying took a toll. In a letter to her mother, she apologized for her worn-down physical appearance. "I'm not fat because I work all day and don't sleep much. I eat a lot. I'm old," she wrote. "I am fifty-five years old and have lived a beautiful and hard life." She developed a stubborn cough. She half-suspected tuberculosis, though her ability to continue working led to doubt. She took paracetamol, ibuprofen, and eventually four rounds of the antibiotic ciprofloxacin, a TB drug, and didn't slow down. Research has since shown that ciprofloxacin can indeed mask the presence of active TB, though of course there is no way of knowing what Annalena was suffering from.

Bishop Giorgio told me, "I take a phrase from the gospel: 'The spirit is willing, but the flesh is weak.' In her, one can say the spirit was keeping up the body. As if the spirit was the driver and the body the poor machine trying to go along. Or, to use an image from here, a donkey cart: the donkey was the spirit and the cart was her body being dragged."

Even the TB center staff teased Annalena about her work ethic. A popular joke started when a staff member told her that if he returned in the morning and still found her at work, he would call Amnesty International and demand Annalena's arrest for violating her own human rights.

If staying in Somaliland wasn't what she wanted, where did Annalena dream of going next? She had no retirement plan and as strongly as she felt pulled to a contemplative life, every time she tried that in Italy, something propelled her back to Africa, back to tuberculosis. Where could she go?

"Sudan," Maria Teresa said.

"Sudan," Shaatos said.

"Sudan," Emanuele Capobianco said.

I met Emanuele in Cesenatico, Italy, where we ate seafood risotto and sipped white wine beside a bay of bright sailboats. Maria Teresa had given me Emanuele's email address one morning in Forlí. A few hours later she called and told me to email Emanuele immediately.

"Tell him Bruno and I support you, otherwise he will never talk with you."

Within minutes of sending my email, Emanuele wrote to schedule our meeting. He said he wouldn't have responded, except for Maria Teresa and Bruno's approval. And he added, "To talk about Annalena is to talk about light, and we can't talk about light without talking about darkness – above all, our own."

I loved his phrasing. The words confirmed what I was experiencing. It was impossible to explore Annalena's life without examining my own. Over lunch, Emanuele said, "No one can talk about Annalena without self-reflection."

Emanuele, who worked at the regional WHO TB office in Cairo at the time, met Annalena in 2001 at a "Tuberculosis in the Third World" conference.

One evening, conference attendees went to a Lebanese restaurant. The table filled with fish, fruit, flat bread, kebabs, and hummus. While he ate, Emanuele spoke with the woman next to him, Annalena.

"She didn't eat a thing," he said. "Just picking, like a bird. She had elegant posture, very regal." Annalena talked about her life and work in Borama with such a "beautiful internal light," Emanuele made a commitment to visit her, which he subsequently did, several times.

With Emanuele, Annalena explored the possibility of moving to Sudan. In September 2001, they decided to take a trip there. They planned to fly out of Nairobi on September 12. After the 9/11 attacks on the United States, Emanuele wondered if they should still go.

"We go," Annalena said.

For two weeks they traveled across southern Sudan. At night they stayed in guest houses and listened to the radio to catch up on world news.

Emanuele learned from Annalena how to assess a TB program. He watched her endless work ethic, her dedication to treating patients properly, and her commitment to seeing nurses well trained.

"We went back to each place two months later," Emanuele said. "She had met dozens of people, but she seemed to remember every single name. We couldn't have spent more than twenty-four hours in a place, but she remembered."

Sudan had nurses, but they weren't trained in adequate TB control. They seemed good-hearted and Annalena had empathy and patience with them. She began to develop a vision of training the nurses in Sudan. With each passing month, as life in Borama became more challenging, she dreamed of Sudan.

They made an effective team. Annalena provided ideas, Emanuele fielded them. They debated the merits, determined what would work best, and Emanuele typed up the notes.

"This led to the first TB guidelines ever in southern Sudan," Emanuele said.

But as much as Annalena struggled in Borama, she could not bring herself to leave, even when Shaatos told her people were losing their affection for her. It was as if, as she had said to Maria Teresa in the train station, God was the one keeping her there and it would take an act of God to pull her away.

Annalena's real trouble began when people stopped responding to treatment. The remarkable 93-percent cure rate she'd had for years, even through the war, plummeted. Now this foreign woman told people they had contagious diseases, and failed to cure them.

When the numbers fell, Annalena brought them to her two most trusted medical advisers, Bruno and Emanuele. Though she had only known Emanuele a short time, Annalena loved him like a son and trusted him implicitly.

"Why are these people not being cured?" she asked. She had already tested for MDR-TB, and Bruno said it was her idea to consider HIV.

Whether it was MDR-TB or HIV, Annalena couldn't cure them. She set aside two rooms at the hospital and one hut outside. The hut was for an MDR-TB patient named Fadouma. The rooms inside were for people with HIV. When they died, locals blamed Annalena.

Emanuele explained how TB programs are evaluated, by a detection rate and treatment success rate. Against a suspected 1,000 cases in a region, how many do you actually find? The target for detecting cases is 75 percent and the target for curing them is 85 percent. Before, Annalena had easily achieved this. When she no longer did, her perfectionist, competitive nature kicked in.

"These numbers don't work anymore," she told Emanuele. "We are masking a big problem and you can't see it with these numbers. I am doing the exact same care and the numbers are going down – people are dying. There must be something more."

"Medically, Annalena was a visionary," Emanuele said. "She was ahead of her time with HIV and MDR-TB because she wasn't just working from the heart, but also with medical knowledge. She matched compassionate care with technical competence, with the highest standards. She pushed the discussion to a different level. If you just looked at the numbers, you would say the center wasn't doing well anymore. It was an interesting moment when numbers said something was wrong, but you couldn't explain why. Even a good public health official could get it wrong, and she was the person who told us this."

He tapped the table with his finger, copying her gestures. "'I know,' she would say, 'I know.'"

Emanuele emphasized the weightiness of this loss of effectiveness. "There was so much pressure on her. And when people started coming and not being cured, that became really dangerous."

In 1997, before she met Emanuele, Annalena had diagnosed her first case of HIV, but she only understood the link between TB and HIV later. People who suspected they were sick with tuberculosis came for treatment, but many had HIV. Within a few years, Annalena saw one or two people with advanced AIDS every day. But the stigma around HIV/AIDS was even stronger than that around TB. As soon as people heard the diagnosis, they fled, or their families took them back, to die in private shame. The few who remained were those who tested positive for both HIV and TB. They could claim they were being treated for TB without mentioning the HIV. At that time, Annalena had almost no way to treat HIV anyway; she could only alleviate symptoms.

HIV scared people. It threatened their lives, their sense of moral superiority, the veracity of their religious beliefs.

"The reason we have HIV," Professor Suleiman said, "is because Borama is close to Ethiopia, so we are more affected." He said HIV came from free sex, illegal sex, and forbidden sex. "Here we have control, not like in Ethiopia. Most of the HIV people are those who bring khat from Ethiopia, traders and drivers."

Based purely on epidemiologic patterns, Professor Suleiman was correct: HIV rates were lower among Muslim populations. However, his words also hinted at more insidious ideas about HIV/AIDS: that because citizens of Borama were Muslim, they were pure and somehow immune to the disease; that free, illegal, and forbidden sex didn't take place in their village; that since having four wives was sanctioned by Islam, HIV wouldn't spread from wife to wife; that conducting an FGM procedure with one blade for multiple girls wouldn't spread the disease.

No one wanted to believe this terrifying scourge had come to their village. Someone had to be blamed and outsiders were the easy target.

"She wants to bring HIV here," people told Shaatos when he went to teashops in town. "She wants to plant it."

"How can she bring AIDS here?" Shaatos said. "People come on their own two legs or relatives bring them here."

Once, the UNHCR donated de-worming pills for children. When Annalena handed out the tablets, people said she was giving out AIDS pills, infecting the children. Another rumor started that she intentionally infected people by reusing syringes. Again, Shaatos defended her. "She uses one-time syringes," he told people. "We have one hundred thousand in stock from the WHO. I keep track of the storage myself. She advises all the nurses to immediately throw away the used needles. I collect them and burn them. I don't bring them somewhere else. I dig a hole, throw it all in, and burn it." He also burned the sputum cups. People knew that, they saw him with the pile of burning detritus. But, he said, they didn't want to believe what their own eyes showed them.

People said Annalena put HIV and tuberculosis in the water. They said she paid people to come to the village and spread the diseases. "They said she wanted to get rid of them," Shaatos said. "They said she was either going to exterminate them or get rich off them. The more sick people she cured, the more famous she would become."

The increasing tension coincided with increasing publicity. In 2001 Annalena presented her testimony at the Vatican. It remains the most extensive, public record of her life, yet afterward she regretted agreeing to what she saw as a spectacle.

The Vatican event was hosted by the Pontifical Council for Health and Ministry to the Sick. "We think Giorgio Bertini put her name in to give testimony," Maria Teresa told me. She was correct. At first, of course, Annalena refused. But the bishop convinced her it was an excellent opportunity. Even her friends in Borama, like Sheikh Saweer of the FGM program, Shaatos, and nurses told her to go. They called it her hajj, her religious pilgrimage.

Publicity also came through visiting journalists. Anna Pozzi was supposed to go to Mogadishu in the summer of 2002, but due to insecurity there she was sent to Borama instead, to interview Annalena.[2]

Annalena met Anna at the door of the TB hospital, and greeted her with a warmth and familiarity that made her feel they'd known each other for years. Annalena provided a quick overview of the work and scanned Anna's clothing. "Better put on a skirt," she said. "That's how women here dress."

Anna hadn't brought a skirt, so Annalena let her borrow one of her own. Though they didn't look alike, they had similar petite body structures, and since she was wearing Annalena's skirt, a rumor began that Anna was her daughter.

"It's useless to deny it," Annalena said, and they both laughed.

Initially, Anna had been disappointed. Mogadishu's stories would have been dramatic. Instead, she found herself with this woman who refused photos and didn't take time to sit for a proper interview. She called it a "disaster, journalistically speaking."

"But Annalena was not a normal person," Anna said later, "and I recognized that right away, not without some discomfort. She was one of those people you meet on the job who change your life in some way. Those who make it a privilege to do this job. The ones who mark you as a person and make you a little different. Maybe a little better.

"And," she added, "you have the impression of being inadequate."

How could any of us measure up to Annalena's standards?

"She made me feel humble," Kitty McKinsey said. "I was in awe of her."

Kitty told Annalena how she felt – that she couldn't do what Annalena did.

Annalena looked at her and said, "But I could not do what you do."

"Annalena made me feel that my choices were as valid as hers," Kitty said. "She was not some kind of saint walking on earth making people feel bad. Her choices were her choices."

Five months after Anna Pozzi left, in November 2002, Annalena contacted her. She said, "As for the article about me – I think it will be better to postpone until after my death, if you still have a sense to publish it. Maybe soon. I could die this very moment."

Her premonition wasn't ill-founded. November and December 2002 would be violent months for expatriates in Somaliland. On December 30, Martin Jutzi, a Swiss businessman who lived in Hargeisa, was shot and killed when he exited the Seven Star grocery store.

For Annalena, the violence had begun with a phone call from Edna Aden in early October. Edna was the former foreign minister of Somaliland and ran a hospital in Hargeisa.

"There is a lady in Hargeisa who is very sick," Edna said. Her name was Roda and she was a former Somalia National Movement guerilla fighter. "Maybe she has HIV. Please, can you check her?"

Edna also suspected tuberculosis and she lacked testing facilities. Annalena agreed to accept Roda. No one in Borama supported her decision, not even her own doctors.

Edna loaded Roda into an ambulance and sent her to Borama. In that one action, the rumors about Annalena were confirmed. She was, indeed, bringing HIV to Borama.

A few weeks later, on October 31, Annalena was in the hospital.

Thud. Thud. Thud. The sound of rocks hitting the roof rattled through the ward. Thud. Thud. More rocks, followed by shouting.

"Death to Annalena!"

Children started throwing the stones, then women, then men.

"We don't want Annalena!"

Even former patients, people cured of TB, shouted for Annalena to leave.

"Death to Annalena!"

Some patients went to the TB center gate and asked what the rioters wanted.

"The woman," they said.

The patients retreated into the clinic. That night Annalena rode in a car to her house a few blocks away, surrounded by armed policemen. The government offered to evacuate her; she laughed at the idea. What hurt her most deeply was that she had to interrupt her treatment of the sick and that the school in the center was accused of spreading Christianity, something Annalena had never engaged in.

Emanuele arrived the next morning and the rock throwing and chanting continued. Annalena was visibly upset, most likely on behalf of her patients, whom the protesters also wanted to kick out of town. But she didn't stop her work. She was tense and shaken, but immovable.

"They do not understand," she said, in a quiet voice. "But the truth can't be stopped. They will understand one day."

The rocks rattled against the roof above her and skidded into the dirt around the wards. The chanting rose above her calm words to the patients. She must have thought back to her early days in Wajir when children threw stones at her and Maria Teresa and called them *galo*. The same grief must have pierced her. Then, being called an infidel. Now, hearing former friends shout for her death. "My story is one of a love rejected," she wrote.[3]

I picture her sitting on the thin mattress, pills in her fingers, a scarf tossed around her gray hair, her eyes gazing at the individual in front of her. She is exhausted but keeping up the fight. It is a bitter moment, one of disappointment and resignation. Yet it marks a turning point, an acceptance of what she has always known: None of us is a hero. We are not even necessary. Life and sickness, goodness and evil, health and hope will continue down the generations. Our life will be poured out here and it might not matter. But if it does make a difference for just one person, that will be enough.

After the riots, Annalena sent an email: "I trust in a resurrection. I let every event settle and rest in the intimate presence of God." She didn't minimize these painful experiences. She fully entered them and let them hurt her because they drew her to God.

Dr. Qaws urged her to place more security guards at her house and the hospital and to hire one to walk her home. She didn't. Dr. Qaws hired his own family members to check on Annalena occasionally and to patrol around her house with weapons after dark. He also went on television to defend Annalena. He called her one of them, a Somali like them. He reminded people of all she had done for their sick and outcast, about the deaf school.

A group of elders visited Annalena at home and told her not to be discouraged. "We are with you," they said. "These people are foolish, and only a few. Most love you."

"But that wasn't true," Shaatos said. "I am Somali; I drank tea in the market and I heard what people said. They were turning against her."

In April 2003 the UNHCR awarded Annalena the prestigious Nansen Refugee Award. Created in 1954, it was named after Fridtjof Nansen, a famous Norwegian polar explorer and the world's first international refugee official. The Nansen is awarded for outstanding service to refugees. Annalena didn't want to accept the award, but it came with a $100,000 prize and she needed the money. She wanted to expand the hospital, to add a physiotherapy department and more rooms for TB patients.

"Money doesn't smell bad," Carlo Astini told me. In other words, take the money and use it. That's what everyone advised her to do. Bishop Giorgio, Shaatos, Bruno, Maria Teresa. Annalena despised what she called "advertising" and praise. When people called her a living legend, when they compared her to Mother Teresa, and when the mayor of Borama awarded her honorary citizenship and named her "person of the year in Somaliland," she said she felt disgusted and ashamed.

But Annalena now had fifty-three staff at the hospital to think of. She bought them all new uniforms every year but had been unable to afford them in 2003. She had 134 inpatients and 137 outpatients, and the number grew every month; in six months she would have almost five hundred. In addition, she paid the school fees for more than seventy children. The deaf school had 263 students, of whom 180 were either orphans or extremely poor. She paid the salaries of the teachers, and salaries for new jobs for the twenty-eight circumcisers who had quit. She needed this money and the publicity, with potentially more funding that would accompany it.

Kitty McKinsey visited Borama with a cameraman to film for the Nansen Award ceremony. The cameraman wanted to film Annalena in her home, sitting on her mattress and eating her pitiful meals of salad, bread, or tea. Annalena wouldn't allow it. Showing her lifestyle and choice of poverty felt exploitative and boastful. Like, from the words of Jesus, letting the left hand know what the right hand was doing.

Since Annalena wouldn't let them film her at home, they followed her to the hospital. While there, the loudspeaker wired through the whole compound sparked to life and a woman's voice came on, extemporaneously creating a poem about Annalena.

Everyone in the compound stopped working and listened, transfixed.

"It was apparently very moving and powerful," Kitty said. "And it went on and on and on. Someone translated a bit for us: a tribute to Annalena and the power of women. Then Annalena came on and thanked the woman and announced that everyone needed to come and take their meds."

Kitty asked Annalena who the poet was.

"The cleaning lady," she said.

"Empowering women was not blah, blah, blah or bureaucracy," Kitty said. "She really did it."

The Nansen Award ceremony was held at the Museé Ariana in Geneva. Annalena was the fifty-ninth recipient of the award. Her mother, Bruno, Enza, Maria Teresa, Roberto, members of the Comitato, and friends traveled to honor her.

Annalena wore a modest gray dress that hung to her ankles, with long sleeves. She tied her hair back in a bun, simple and elegant. She gave a moving speech to a packed audience. The room was warm and several people fanned themselves with their programs, but Annalena showed no sign of heat or sweat. Neither did Maria Teresa, who gazed at Annalena from her seat, her eyes bright with affection.

Annalena returned to Borama in July 2003 without the award money. Geneva was slow to process it. She had no bank account in Somaliland; Bishop Giorgio managed her account in Djibouti. The funds remained tied up in bureaucracy for weeks. And then months. She also returned to Borama exposed to fame, giving fuel to the rumor that she only helped the sick for her own benefit. Villagers realized how much power this woman had, as the mooryan had discovered in Merka.

In August, Annalena wrote in an email, "I am ever in need. The $100,000 of Nansen are tied up. And they can only be used for building and for long-lasting equipment."[4] She couldn't give the money as salaries or gifts, as much as her staff would have preferred that.

Annalena allocated the Nansen money for a physiotherapy center attached to the administration building. It was to be built in three stages and handed over to the local authorities for management on Monday, October 6, 2003, before completion of the structure.

The Borama Hospital Authority gave Annalena a twenty-by-sixty-foot plot of land near the hospital mosque for the building. Later, when the building was completed, the entrance was only four yards from the mosque entrance. One report commented that "it could not be established whether the mosque was part of the hospital or if the hospital was encroaching upon it." This proximity made people nervous. She put TB and HIV right at the doorstep of a place of worship and prayer.

Deciding how to eventually hand over the building to the local authorities had been complicated, and Annalena claimed the problem was greed. Because of the Nansen Award, people assumed the hospital was a source of wealth. Even though everything Annalena did in her own life pointed to the opposite, some people thought she had bags full of cash at her house and at the hospital.

"Nansen was a turning point," Emanuele said. "It stressed her out and put her in the limelight." He visited in September 2003. "I don't think I've ever been as in tune with her as that afternoon," he said. "The last words of a person are like a legacy. We talked about the struggle with the community, the struggle to defend the least. I told her, life is so quick."

"Live it to the fullest," Annalena told him, and hugged him goodbye.

"Her eyes were clear. She knew she was in danger."

HIV was a broiling issue. Annalena's emails reveal more of the pressures she was under: "The struggle here is enormous. I fear the staff will burst and eventually rebel. Patients, many of them, seem able to talk only of their desire to infect us and to commit suicide. It is more and more clear that only hope of being cured, which only antiretroviral drugs may offer, will be able to change the situation and give way to a positive relationship with sufferers. . . . The fact is that I am quite alone. . . . Forgive me if I sound harsh. Believe me, my heart is bleeding."

Annalena received a death threat. Bishop Giorgio took a photocopy of the first one. Then the second one. A sheikh in Borama preached against Annalena and said the infidel should be killed. A Somaliland newspaper published a cartoon of Annalena. It depicted a white woman, her face sober, her eyes tired, and her body weary. Around her neck hung a box with the Somaliland School for the Deaf inside and an eye on the wall with two tears dripping down. With both hands, she held over her head the brick-walled Borama TB Hospital and on top of the hospital is a line of skeletons, holding their heads and tucking their faces into their knees.

Dr. Qaws urged her to leave.

"No," she told him. "I will stay here. I will even die here."

As Dr. Walhad later said about the conversation between Annalena and Dr. Qaws, "She decided."

On September 18 Annalena wrote, "These are months of persecution. I'm a lamb led to the slaughter. I am at the center of a violent movement, all darkness and evil, a witch-hunt. There is denial of truth, justice, compassion, and love. My fight for good, forgiveness, truth, justice, compassion, and liberation is tougher than ever, hindered by the forces of evil. Do not worry! See you soon, God willing."[5]

On October 3, she wrote, "I am under tremendous trials. But, all courage. All strength. All light."

As Emanuele said, one's last words are a legacy. These are among the last emails Annalena wrote.

In early 2003, on the road from Hargeisa to Gabiley, at the turnoff to Ethiopia, police stopped a taxi. They searched the vehicle and found piles of cash, Ethiopian biir, in the trunk. A vicious firefight followed, and the occupants of the taxi escaped. One of them was Ahmed Abdi Godane.

When Godane and the others fled into the desert, no one pursued them. The taxi, the bales of biir, even the gunfight, had little meaning to the police at the time. Maybe it had been a robbery, maybe it was a khat payment or an illegal currency exchange. In retrospect, after Godane was identified as the leader of the group that would become al-Shabaab, it showed how desperate Godane and his followers were. Unorganized, poorly funded, haphazardly structured, the would-be terrorists, some of whom had recently returned from Saudi Arabia and Afghanistan, relied on hijackings and theft. What they needed was a consolidating act, an event that proved to a global jihadi network that they were serious and capable. Only then could they form a more official and respected terror organization. Only then would they receive help from abroad in the form of more sophisticated weapons and fighters.

They started to hunt for a target.

17

Legacy

AMINA WAS AT HOME with her husband. Shaatos was at home with his wife, Salwa, his mother, and his eldest son. Koos, a nursing student from Edna Aden's hospital, was in the TB hospital compound. I was in my house in Borama, watching a movie.

Annalena was on the ground, bleeding into the dirt.

The shooter sprinted away under cover of darkness. Koos and her coworker, Khush, heard the shot. Koos thought it was a stone hitting one of the water tanks outside the ward they had just exited. Patients inside thought the same thing and didn't get out of bed, not right away. Koos turned around. She saw Annalena on the ground and froze. Khush ran toward Annalena. He saw the blood and shouted that he would get help. He sprinted to the general hospital, just on the other side of the clearing and returned with two doctors.

Koos emerged from her shock as they moved Annalena into the hospital. Nothing made sense. Koos hadn't seen anyone, hadn't heard any conversation or argument, only the metallic bang. Annalena made no sound, no shout or cry. From the front she didn't even appear injured. Just a little blue spreading under the skin of her forehead. Koos didn't want to see the back of Annalena's head, the exit wound.

Did Annalena have time to see the man's face before he pulled the trigger? Did she have time to realize this was how it would all end?

Shaatos saw people running. Children, then a woman, then a man. Running. He called outside, "What happened?"

"Don't you know?" someone shouted back. "Your mother was killed."

"What? Who?"

"Annalena."

Shaatos started to run toward the hospital.

A woman ran to Amina's house. She gestured that Annalena had been shot. Amina didn't believe her. She and her husband walked toward the hospital. They saw commotion. Doctors, lines of people. Amina started to run.

Fifteen minutes after the shot, while Amina and Shaatos were still running, Borama police arrested two men. Mustafa Mohamed Yusuf, known as Ali, and Abibaker Mohamed Ismail. Someone claimed to have overheard Mustafa threatening Annalena earlier that afternoon. He said she would be in trouble if she didn't give him the job of driver. Annalena didn't promise him the job. She couldn't because, so far, the hospital had no money to purchase the intended vehicle.

Amina reached Annalena before Shaatos. She remembers blood. Blood on Annalena, blood on the ground, the line of people who wanted to donate blood. Shaatos arrived and pushed his way through the crowd.

"*Ubannee*," he shouted as he ran, "Move." The people made an open space for him. He held Annalena's head. Her eyes fluttered, and she gasped a few times. "I held her for almost twenty minutes and she was struggling. She was dying. She was so full of blood. Rachel, you can't imagine. Pools of blood. They tried to replace the blood she lost, that was the only thing they could do."

Dr. Qassim, a Somali doctor who worked with Annalena in southern Somalia and was in Borama at the time, telephoned Bruno. "Annalena was shot down," he said. "She is in the hospital. We don't know what to do."

Drs. Qaws and Walhad brought Annalena to Borama's primary hospital, which shared a wall with the TB center. But the hospital had almost no equipment and there was nothing the doctors could do except try to stop the bleeding and replace the lost blood. The doctors finally stood back.

"Shaatos," they said, "we did our best. We can't save her."

"What do we do?" Shaatos said. "What do we do?"

Annalena stopped breathing. Shaatos started to weep. Dr. Qassim moved him away from Annalena. Dr. Qassim called Bruno again.

"It was 9:00 p.m.," Bruno remembered.

Dr. Qassim told Bruno his sister was dead. "What should we do with her body?" Qassim asked.

"Please take her to Nairobi," Bruno said.

He, Enza, and Maria Teresa boarded a plane that night, heading for Kenya.

Zahara, from the FGM group, entered the room with another nurse. The two women washed Annalena's body and wrapped it in a white cloth, the Muslim tradition. They tied strings on her ankles and her waist, over the white shroud, and put her body into an ambulance. They closed the door.

"I stood there," Shaatos said. "It was night. My heart was broken."

Dr. Abdirahman Jama Had, the regional medical officer, wrote Annalena's death certificate.

"The inlet of the bullet was observed at the left frontal bone and the outlet was seen at the occipital bone. . . . After intensive care and proper re-animations like blood transfusions, IV fluids, and oxygen therapy, Annalena Tonelli expired at 9:00 p.m. in Borama Regional Hospital."

Koos stayed with Annalena until long after midnight, still traumatized. But when she came out of the hospital, the police were waiting for her, and for Khush. The two nurses were arrested as suspects, perhaps accomplices. They were held for two days, then taken to court. The court found nothing against them and they were released. The two men who had argued and been arrested were also eventually released. Koos hurried to Hargeisa, to her mother, away from death. But less than twenty-four hours later, she would be back in Borama, back at the job she would hold for the next fifteen years, carrying on Annalena's work.

I knew nothing until the next morning. My housekeeper provided the first clue something had happened when she told me Annalena had been struck. Or, at least that was how I interpreted her words. I couldn't fathom she meant Annalena had been killed. I called my coworker, Martha Erickson. Both of our husbands taught at Amoud University and there was no cell phone coverage there. Martha said Annalena had been shot and our husbands were being escorted back to our houses. She had also been in touch with our boss, in Hargeisa.

"He ordered us to Hargeisa," Martha said. "We'll stay maybe all day, maybe two days. There is a safe apartment at Edna Aden's hospital."

I packed a bag for one night. When my husband came home, we drove the two hours to the capital.

On Monday, October 6 at 5:50 a.m. Bishop Giorgio said a requiem Mass for Annalena in Mogadishu and boarded a Daallo Airlines flight to Hargeisa.

Bishop Giorgio kept a detailed journal of his three days in Hargeisa and he wrote out the questions everyone was asking. What will happen to the TB program without her? The school for the deaf? The anti-FGM campaign? HIV awareness, promotion of women, funding for the new physiotherapy building? The blind school, school fees, salaries for the four deaf Somali teachers from Kenya? The tailoring teacher? Who would fund the laboratory?

Shaatos told him of a meeting among the TB clinic staff; all had promised to continue the work, a promise they have kept. Koos, the laundry workers and kitchen staff, Zahara, Sheikh Saweer – they all still work at the TB clinic or with other projects initiated by Annalena.

The bishop wanted to celebrate a public Mass, but the officer in charge of security for the UN and international NGOs decided it was too risky. Ten people gathered in a home. Someone pulled out a secret bottle of wine from Italy, the bishop had the wherewithal to write down the name, Valpolicella, and with an English Bible, a French Bible, and an Italian Missal, they celebrated the Eucharist together.

I wonder if, in the back of his mind, the bishop was thinking about the crumbs of bread in Annalena's house, the body of Christ, now behind enemy lines with no one to protect it. Later, he would send Father Sandro to search Annalena's house. The house remained untouched because, as Shaatos said, everyone knew she owned nothing. Father Sandro found the bread in a satchel hanging on a nail inside Annalena's wooden wardrobe and consumed it.

The day my family and our coworkers were supposed to spend in Hargeisa extended to seven days. I brought a handful of diapers, one change of clothes, and only two books. Our apartment was furnished with two mattresses and a table with four chairs. We were seven people. We ate spaghetti from the market with our fingers, out of plastic bags. We played endless games of "Ring around the Rosy" with our three toddlers. We tried not to yell at each other out of boredom, stress, or fear. And finally, we pleaded with our boss to allow us to return to Borama. We would be careful; we would hire extra armed guards; the men would use an escort to and from the university; the women wouldn't go outside the house. We didn't expect these measures to last long. Either life would return to normal or we would leave the country. Life under lockdown wasn't the kind of life we wanted.

On October 13, we drove back to Borama. In the car, we talked about Annalena. We didn't believe the rumors Somalis believed – we knew she didn't give children AIDS pills or come to Borama to get rich. But looking back now, I can see we had our own set of misconceptions based on bias and ignorance.

"She was Catholic," someone in the car said.

"Was she a nun?" I asked. Unmarried, Catholic – must be a nun.

"No, she wasn't a nun, she just never married." At the time, I didn't know why – that she loved the desert, the poor, and Jesus, and this was enough.

"Was she a missionary?" I asked.

No. Yes. What is a missionary? If a missionary is a person supported financially by a religious organization with the intention of evangelizing and teaching people about Jesus and the Bible, she wasn't. If a missionary is a person who serves the poor and hopes to have a positive impact on the world, because of Jesus, she probably was.

Was she a martyr or a victim? A victim's death is referred to in the context of the cause of death – a victim of cancer, a victim of violence. A martyr's death is referred to in the context of the cause she lived for – a martyr for peace, for justice, for faith. If Annalena was a victim, her death was a tragedy. If she was a martyr, her death was an inspiration, a sacrifice, an honor.

"Was she a Christian?" I asked. The car was silent.

Yes, at the time I was *that* kind of Christian. Now I look back at this conversation and my arrogance and spiritual legalism and feel ashamed. Jesus told his disciples that the people around them would know who they were by their love. If I had paid any attention to Annalena's love, I never would have asked that question. Annalena loved Jesus and acted more like him than anyone I've ever known. Compared to this, these other labels – Catholic, nun, missionary, martyr, victim, Christian – are irrelevant. The thing that counts is love.

News of Annalena's murder zipped around the world. UNHCR Goodwill Ambassador Angelina Jolie wrote, "Dr. Annalena, the Italian aid worker, was shot point blank while attending her patients in Somalia. For over twenty-five years, she lived and worked benevolently in East Africa, where she established free health clinics." [1]

Many of the reports and news articles were sprinkled with inaccuracies. Annalena was not a doctor. She was not a nun, though that was a common assumption. She worked for thirty-four years in Somalia and Kenya. She did far more than establish free health clinics. Who *was* she? What *did* she do? Would the world ever find out?

Ruud Lubbers, the High Commissioner of the UNHCR, was told of her death on the telephone. He was silent a long time and then said, "Now they start killing the angels." [2]

The Tuesday after her death, her fellow Nansen Award winners wrote an open letter condemning the murder: "We are far from deluding ourselves that humanitarian work can be done without risks, but these must be within reason. Otherwise aid workers will become extinct and the people they serve will be left to their own resources."

I understand the point of this letter. Humanitarians have increasingly become intentional targets in conflict areas. Annalena would decry the violence against aid workers, but I don't think she would mind if a certain kind of humanitarian became extinct, the kind she bristled against her entire career. If someone was prepared to sacrifice, unafraid of the increasing risks, she would welcome that.

Also, it might not be as terrible as Westerners imagine for people to be left to their own resources. Annalena used to bring a water truck to supply the deaf school. After her death, the town donated water pipes. After her death, the local electrical company agreed to provide free electricity to the school. The food preparation she oversaw at her home moved directly into the hospital and a kitchen facility was built, with local funding. Her guard, Rashid, got a job at the hospital. In other words, the resources were available. It is never true that without humanitarians, people have no resources. What Borama needed, and what Annalena provided, beyond access to some specific resources, was knowledge and hope. Her example inspired people to move forward on their own.

On the Tuesday after her death, Borama's mayor addressed a crowd of five thousand. He said the town would name a street after Annalena and establish a memorial. That Friday during prayer time, imams in more than thirty mosques in Borama expressed condolences and condemned Annalena's murder.

The same newspaper that printed the earlier cartoon printed another. This one showed Annalena, again with her hair covered, listening to a child's lungs with a stethoscope. The child is hunched over, and he says, "Uncle, just today let her go. Let her heal me first." Behind Annalena is a bearded man pointing a handgun at the back of her head. In the background is a row of TB patients, lying in beds. The man says,

"In Burco and in Hargeisa the infidels were killed." At the muzzle of the gun is a small word, "Bub." He shot her.

In Forlí, twenty-five hundred people attended Mass at the Cathedral Santa Croce, spilling into the street, many of them in tears. Two hundred people came to the Consolata Shrine in Nairobi for a memorial service. Italian President Carlo Azeglio Ciampi gave a speech, honoring Annalena. He also gave the Comitato a medal in her memory. Ivano Natali, then president of the Comitato, said, "This medal should serve as a stimulus to continue her work. . . . However, it would have been better to help Annalena, and listen to her, when she was alive."

While Emanuele waited for Bruno, Enza, and Maria Teresa's plane to land, he went to Wilson Airport to meet Annalena's body.

Airport employees unloaded the simple wooden coffin. Someone in Hargeisa had carefully placed a cross on top of the coffin. Emanuele found the gesture moving, knowing a Muslim had placed it there. By the time the body arrived, the cross had shifted and was crooked, so he nudged it straight again. Along with the coffin, someone packed a few of Annalena's belongings – a Bible, pieces of paper, two dresses, sandals that had been a gift from a patient, a scarf from the staff, and books.

"Our last encounter was very positive," Emanuele said. "There was closure in the sense that she had the life she wanted. She wished this would be her end, to give her life for something. So that gave me a lot of peace and an immense sense of gratitude that allows me to see this as a life well lived, fully lived."

Emanuele delivered her body to the morgue, then met the plane from Italy.

Catholic leaders in Italy wanted Bruno to send Annalena's body back to Forlí. There could be a public feast, a religious funeral. She would become known and famous all over Italy, maybe all over the world.

"But she didn't want this," Bruno said.

They decided to cremate Annalena in Nairobi and carried the ashes by plane to Wajir. Bruno brought a small plaque for which Enza had chosen this inscription: "The lame will walk, the blind will see. The desert will flourish."

Bruno, Enza, Maria Teresa, and Emanuele, joined in Wajir by Elmi and Kali, placed the plaque inside the hermitage and scattered Annalena's ashes.

They returned the same day to Nairobi. Another shipment had arrived with a few more of Annalena's books and her final will. In the will, she wrote that she wished to be cremated and the ashes scattered in Wajir, in the hermitage.

Maria Teresa sighed. "That was a fantastic moment, when we discovered we had done just what she wanted."

A white tile pillar on top of a rough cement base was built in the exact place Annalena was killed. The base is a crooked square, the corners rounded where chips of cement have broken off. The cement is uneven in tone, with large, dark blotches. The pillar stands approximately ten feet high and some of the tiles used were broken and glued together, giving the pillar the look of a patchwork quilt. On one side there is an open area of cement where words were carved while the cement was still wet. The letters were written with the quality of a child scrawling an afterthought with his finger.

TB

Started

24/11/1996

To

5 Oct 2003

There is no mention of Annalena by name or of the events surrounding her death. There is no tender message or epitaph, no recollection of the years she spent in southern Somalia or Kenya. Nothing about HIV, FGM, schools for the deaf and blind, the orphans she raised. It is as if Annalena herself were never there.

Epilogue

ON OCTOBER 22, 2003, Richard and Enid Eyeington sat down in their living room in Sheikh, Somaliland, to watch TV. The British couple in their mid-sixties taught at an SOS Kinderdorf boarding school in a small village a few hours from Borama.

They were shot through the window.

The next morning the Eyeingtons' housekeeper found the front door locked. She forced her way inside. Richard and Enid still sat in their chairs, dead. Bullet holes punctured the wall across from the window, and the television was smashed. Nothing had been stolen.

Claudio Croce, the Eyeingtons' coworker with SOS based in Nairobi, received a phone call that morning with the news. Claudio chartered a plane and landed in Hargeisa that afternoon. SOS staff sent the bodies to a morgue in Hargeisa, where Claudio had to identify them. Richard was filled with bullet wounds, but recognizable. Enid's body and face had been so destroyed, Claudio had nightmares for months.

The SOS community was shocked. There had been no hint, no threats, no previous violence. There seemed to be no clear motive. The Eyeingtons were simply teachers.

The broader expatriate community in Somaliland was also shocked, and whether or not one of the motives behind these murders was to get rid of the foreigners, that is what happened. Everyone left. The Red Cross, the UN, the EU, NGOs. My family.

I got a phone call around ten o'clock in the morning on October 23. It was our boss in Hargeisa. He had just returned from an official security meeting.

"Get Tom home from the university," he said. "He needs to come home now."

I didn't like the fear I heard in his voice.

"Two teachers were shot and killed last night."

Teachers. We were teachers. What if someone was coming after us?

I couldn't reach Tom on the phone. I didn't know what to do. I paced and prayed. An hour later he drove through the front gate. I almost cried.

At noon, we got another phone call. "Leave. Now. You're booked on a flight that leaves Hargeisa at 2:00."

Hargeisa was a two-hour drive; even if we left that instant, we would miss it. But we threw a suitcase and a backpack into the car, grabbed the twins, and left. I didn't go back to Borama for fourteen years.

I asked everyone I interviewed three questions about Annalena's death. How did they hear the news? What would they speculate as to motive? Were they surprised? The last question was the easiest. No one was surprised.

Shaatos refused to speculate beyond saying the intention was to get rid of all the foreigners, the *galo*, the infidel.

Roberto said Bruno called him. As to motive? "Let us not speak of death. Let us speak of life."

Antonio said his wife Monica told him. She heard about it on TV and called him.

"He started to cry," she said.

"So much emotion," Antonio said, in Italian, but the words were clear.

Carlo Astini and Miriam Martinelli, now married, worked at the Italian Hospital in Balbala, Djibouti. Carlo said, "Someone from the hospital told me an Italian was shot in Somaliland. Somalis knew right away. But for me, she couldn't die. She was eternal because of the faith she had." He paused and swallowed hard. "Even if I didn't see her often, I am still moved thinking of her."

Amina had four ideas regarding motive. She mentioned the driver who wanted a job. "But she didn't need a car. So, two – a doctor wanted to kick her out of town. Or, three – people were corrupt. Or, four – a fight over a new x-ray room." I suspected she meant the physiotherapy building. I had also heard a rumor that people were angry this building came so close to the mosque.

Kamu, a German journalist in Kenya, suggested her murder was connected to the Wagalla Massacre. In January 2003, Mike Harries, the pilot and windmill builder, had come to Borama and, through tears, pleaded with Annalena to testify in Kenya. The government had finally opened an investigation, a Truth, Justice, and Reconciliation Committee, and now was the time for Annalena to tell her story for the legal and public record. She wouldn't do it. She said that time of her life was finished. And now, according to Kamu, her version of events would never be fully known, a great relief to high-level Kenyan politicians.

Elmi was convinced the murder had been planned and committed by precursors to today's al-Shabaab terrorist group, to create fear among foreigners.

"A driver could not do this," he said, rejecting the theory of the man who wanted a job. "Look at the way it was planned. If it was a local, it would have come out so easily, the people would have known, the nurses would recognize him. They are more spontaneous: you offend me, I kill you. But these people planned it. It was Islamic groups." He made good points. "And, if it was just a stupid driver, no one would hide it from you. But people didn't want to talk. This means it was someone else."

Antoinette saw Annalena's death in terms of the eternal battle between good and evil. "In the world if I love you, I expect something back. It is difficult to love freely. But the true love is to give freely, to give, give, give. This kind of love she gave to everybody, Somalis good and bad. It brought her to death because that kind of love is impossible."

Bishop Giorgio is convinced Annalena is a martyr. He used the technical term, *in odium fidei*, which meant she was killed out of hatred for her Christian faith. "For radical Muslims, her presence was a constant slap in the face," he said. "She was a real human religious person. They were pretending to be truly religious but she, without pretending anything, was really motivated by faith. True religion, helping the poor. This could be why she was killed."

Somaliland's President Dahir Riyale Kahin told journalist Maggie Black that the murder was part of a deliberate effort to destabilize the north and to force it to rejoin southern Somalia.

But then, with one further conversation as I wrapped up research for this book, the mystery of who killed Annalena morphed into a different mystery. Matt Bryden, a Canadian security and terrorism investigator and journalist, was adamant: her murderer had confessed and was in prison in Hargeisa.

Why, then, would no one admit the murder had been solved? Why would no one talk about the confessed murderer?

I understood why Annalena's family didn't want to talk about the case – they chose to focus on her life. I understood why people who weren't intimately involved at the end of her life, like Carlos and Miriam, hadn't heard news reports from Somaliland. But surely Somalis in Somaliland knew the case was solved.

There was a lot of confusion after the Eyeingtons were murdered, Bryden said. No connections were made, yet, but foreigners evacuated Somaliland. Then, in 2004, a car driving between Hargeisa and Berbera stopped to help two women stranded by a broken-down vehicle. When the car stopped, the women threw off their hijabs, revealing themselves to be armed men, and fired into the car. A Kenyan woman, Florence Cheruiyot, was killed, and a German man was shot through the neck, though he would survive. The driver summoned the courage to drive away. The attackers fled.

While the driver sped away, he called the police. A bulletin was sent out to the surrounding villages to look for a red Toyota Surf. The attackers were captured in Togashe, near the Ethiopian border.

Implicated in this attack, Godane and other leaders such as al-Afghani escaped to Mogadishu. There, forced into close quarters, they began to plan another attack, this time targeting Somaliland President Kahin's children. An informant tipped the president off to the plan and Somaliland police were on high alert.

The group of aspiring terorrists arrived in Hargeisa in 2005 and took a taxi from the airport to a house, their base of operations. The taxi driver grew suspicious because of the large and unusually heavy luggage the men carried, and reported it to the police. The police decided to launch a raid. They quietly surrounded the house and then, for reasons that remain unclear, opened fire.

Chaos ensued as the policemen fired through the house, hitting policemen on the opposite side. Some of the occupants were injured, others escaped. One of the would-be escapees was injured and captured before he could disappear into the bush. "This is the man who shot Annalena," Bryden said. "He admitted to pulling the trigger."

This man was Abdirahman Mohamed Jaama, known as Indo-adhe. He was from Borama, a member of the town's primary clan, the Gedhabuursi.

Also captured was Ahmed Ali Issa, the sniper who killed Richard and Enid Eyeington.

"They know," Bryden said of the local authorities. "But Annalena was killed before the police were ready to admit that this problem existed. If you say this happened, you have to look into your own family and it is there, too."

It is far easier to blame the murder on a mentally unstable man or on Annalena's own naivete about AIDS, TB, and FGM, than to admit the festering of a violent fundamentalist strain in one's own family, village, or nation.

Annalena was one of the first foreign victims of the groups that would become al-Shabaab. Killing her, and then the Eyeingtons, provided Godane and the others the confidence they needed to raise money and organize. They needed to make a big show, to prove they weren't *fadhi-dil*, fighting from a sitting position. It worked. Al-Shabaab pulled off the Nairobi Westgate Mall attack in 2013, a suicide bomb attack in Djibouti in 2014, and the attack on a university in Garissa in 2015.

Annalena was a soft target, and a high-profile one. The knowledge that her murder was a precursor to al-Shabaab was unsettling for me. Like Somalilanders, I preferred to think of the killing as targeting her work or her money. This, the need for any victim, meant it could have been my husband. Or me. Or our whole family.

"Why not us?" I asked my husband.

"We were a little bit harder," he said.

One of the first trainings we received before moving to Somaliland taught us to make ourselves a "harder target." Just a little harder than the person next to you. I hated the thought, because it meant putting someone else at risk, making survival a cruel competition. But Annalena didn't care. She knew she was a soft target. She refused weapons at the hospital, didn't like them at her house, insisted on staying out after dark. We never left the house after dark, and our guard had a weapon. Those small choices may have made a difference; I will likely never know.

"It doesn't matter who killed her," Bruno said. "What matters is that she is not here anymore."

"But she is still present," Enza said quietly. "We feel her, more than when she was alive."

In 2015, I sat in a conference room in the Catholic cathedral in Djibouti. High ceilings and long, narrow windows kept the room cool. I flipped through letters, emails, photographs, and newspaper clippings Bishop Giorgio had kept. In one manila folder I came upon an email from a group monitoring and connecting international NGOs in Somaliland.

The email said the UN was evacuating all staff and recommended NGOs follow suit. The printout included all the "sent to" addresses and among them was the address of our boss. This was the email that forced the end of our dream of working in Somalia and, possibly, saved our lives.

It was also the intersection between Annalena's life and my own. The thought settled over me like a mantle. I had never met her, but twelve years earlier her death had dramatically reshaped the rest of my life. I had never intended to live in

Djibouti and now I have been here since 2004. If that were the only impact, it would have felt significant enough. But now that I knew Annalena and had met her family and run my fingers over notes she scribbled in prayer books and wrapped her blanket around my shoulders, I knew she had changed me in far more profound ways.

I came into her story with the idea that Annalena was a development worker with a Christian identity. I now saw she was both and neither. She did development work but not like anyone else I knew. If forced to choose a religious label, Christian would be the best fit, but she eschewed labels all her life. She was a woman who loved Jesus and who loved the poor, and she was a woman for whom love was not an emotion, it was an action. The same can be said about her faith. As Antoinette said, if faith is love, Annalena had a mountain.

Annalena could be simplistically presented as a saint. That is what some in the Catholic Church would like. But it's the last thing the people who loved Annalena want. On the tenth anniversary of her death a priest told Bruno that she should be beatified. "It will take time," the priest said, "but we will do it."

"I would prefer if he said, 'No. Never,'" Bruno said. "As long as we live we will not let that happen. We don't want to make her into an Annalena that she never was. She was a saint. But to make her a church saint and put her on an altar and forget her? No."

"She doesn't belong to the church," Maria Teresa said. "She belongs to the poor. My constant concern is to show what was human in her. To put her in a Catholic saint box would be to limit her."

Even the comparison to Mother Teresa falls short.

"She was not a Mother Teresa of Somalis," Emanuele said. "Mother Teresa accompanied people to death too, but less with the idea of curing them. Annalena really was there to save them. She spent nights holding dying people, yes. But her service was aimed at improving the dignity and quality of life, not just the dignity and quality of death."

Service ultimately comes down to love, and love is as simple and as distressing as holding a dying person's hand or bringing a cup of cold water to a tuberculosis patient. Simple, because anyone can do it. Distressing, because most of us wish we could do so much more. We want to be world changers and it is hard to admit we are weak, only strong enough to love one person at a time. Annalena proves that love in action is simple, yes. But it is also profound enough to truly change the world.

Maria Teresa said it best. "Annalena is a universal figure and a universal way of religion because she belongs to the religion of love. Raised as a Catholic in a Catholic family and country. Behaved as a Somali and a Muslim in Africa. Died and then cremated as a Hindu, disappearing into fire and wind. If God exists, he is a God of love. Annalena is universal because love is universal."

Acknowledgments

THIS BOOK WOULD NOT EXIST without the vision and drive of Matt Erickson, videographer and researcher extraordinaire. Thank you for working with me all these years.

Bruno, Enza, and Maria Teresa, receiving your support in telling this story is one of the great honors of my life. Thank you for opening your hearts, homes, and memories – for sharing Annalena with the world.

To everyone else who spoke with me, helped with translations and medical research, hosted me, and believed this book was important, thank you. You shared your sorrows and joys, answered endless questions, introduced me to *stroopwafel*, taught me how to eat Italian pizza, bought me a toothbrush, and made a firecracker birthday cake for my mother. Listening to your stories has been a profound privilege. I am, I hope, a better and braver and more loving person because of each of you:

Andrea Saletti, Francesca Saletti, Eleonora Saletti, Annalena Saletti, Luciano Saletti, Viviana Tonelli, Mila, Antonio and Monica Gabrielli, Roberto Gimelli, Mario Neri, Emanuele Capobianco, Dr. Qaws, Dr. Walhad, Shaatos and Salwa, the Van der Poel family, Amina Mohamed Dahiye, Abdullahi Italianiga, Bishop Giorgio Bertin, Antoinetta, Father Sandro,

Carlo Astini, Miriam Martinelli, Claudio Croce, Father Tom, Elmi Ibrahim, Bishar Ismacil Ibrahim, Zahra and Mohamed, Hussein Mohamed Ahmed, Kali Mohamed Abdi, Suleiman Ahmed Gulaid, Senator Abdirahman, Sister Terizia Goynyokarada, Marcie Gowan, Kitty McKenzie, Sister Marzia, Luca Vitali, Akihiro Seita, Marina Madeo, Liddia Maggi, Ariana, Serena, Anna Cataldi, Anna Pozzi, Dr. Firdosi Mehta, Matt Bryden, Mike Harries, Fathia, Ivano Natali, Silvio Tessari, Massimo Orlandi, Dr. Abdi Aziz Oskar, Dr. Sara, Dr. Kara, Dr. Mohamed, Koos, Edna Aden, Hassan Kow Mumin, Nuura, Sheikh Saweer Mohamed, Maaho, Khalad'la, Nik Ripken, Scott and Sharon Karstenson, Dr. Peter Bird, Dr. Jon Fielder, Dr. Annie Mikobi, Dr. Kelly Pieh, Stephanie and Shoshon Tamasweet, Kevin Pieh, Nancy Njoki, Abdillahi Lab Dheere, Martha Erickson.

Thank you to all the anonymous people who helped me find books at libraries or catch trains, who hunted down obscure documents in archives or watched out for my safety. Your generosity and kindness are what makes the world a lovely place to explore.

To the editing and publishing team at Plough, your support and encouragement have been invaluable in bringing Annalena's story to the world. Thank you for welcoming me at the Bruderhof, where you choose the path of radical love, hope, and faith. Special thanks to my editor Sam Hine, Sarah Hine, Trevor Wiser, and Maureen Swinger.

Lyla Taddei, Marilyn Gardner, Hannah Cowell: cheerleaders, email readers, wise advisors, thank you for your friendship. Thank you to the writing community of Hope Writers, too many to name. Ken and Barb Pieh, Mom and Dad, one of you offered insightful editing suggestions and one of you offered tears. Thank you for always, always being there for me.

Thank you Magdalene, Henry, and Lucy, for letting Mom travel and work and fill our living room with index cards and stacks of books, for listening to me talk about Annalena too much, and for generally making my life beautiful.

Thank you, Tom, for believing in me more than I do. You are my best decision. We have seen the world together and we haven't found them yet, but one day we will discover dragons.

Notes

1. The Tuberculosis Holy Grail

1. Chana Gazit, director, *The Forgotten Plague*, PBS, American Experience, air date February 10, 2015.
2. More recently called the North Eastern Province.
3. Abjata Khalif, "TB Stigma Fuels Gender Violence," The African Woman and Child Feature Service (AWC).
4. Christian W. McMillen, *Discovering Tuberculosis: A Global History, 1900 to the Present* (New Haven: Yale University Press, 2015), 68.
5. McMillen, *Discovering Tuberculosis*, 126.
6. Wajir Tuberculosis Project, typed document from Bruno Tonelli.
7. McMillen, *Discovering Tuberculosis*, 10.
8. McMillen, *Discovering Tuberculosis*, 10.

2. Ghandi and a Prostitute

1. Annalena Tonelli to Bruno Tonelli, July 10, 1969, in *Lettere dal Kenya*, B. Tonelli, E. Tonelli, M. Battistini (Bologna: EBD, 2016).
2. Annalena Tonelli, November 2, 1982, in *Lettere dal Kenya*.
3. Pope Paul VI, *Apostolicam actuositatem*, November 18, 1965.
4. David Brown, "A Breath of Fresh Air," *Washington Post*, February 24, 1993.
5. Annalena Tonelli to Maria Teresa Battistini, August 29, 1982, in *Lettere dal Kenya*.

3. Desert Paradise

1. Derek Franklin, *A Pied Cloak* (London: Janus Publishing Company, 2007), 111.
2. Franklin, *A Pied Cloak*.
3. Douglas Jardine, *The Mad Mullah of Somaliland* (London: H. Jenkins, 1923), 122.
4. Annalena Tonelli to Guido Tonelli, May 13, 1972, in *Lettere dal Kenya*.
5. Annalena Tonelli, in *Lettere dal Kenya*.
6. Annalena Tonelli to Guido Tonelli, May 7, 1972, in *Lettere dal Kenya*.
7. Annalena Tonelli to "Beloved," March 9, 1970, in *Lettere dal Kenya*.
8. Annalena Tonelli to "Beloved," March 9, 1970, in *Lettere dal Kenya*.

4. Thirst

1. Elspeth Huxley, *Out in the Midday Sun* (Vintage Digital, 2011), Chapter 12.
2. Margaret Laurence, *The Prophet's Camel Bell: A Memoir of Somaliland*, (University of Chicago Press, reprint, 2012), 53.

5. Infidel

1. Annalena Tonelli, April 17, 1970, in *Lettere dal Kenya.*
2. Annalena Tonelli, April 26, 1970, in *Lettere dal Kenya.*
3. Annalena Tonelli, October 1, 1972, in *Lettere dal Kenya.*
4. Annalena Tonelli, *Vatican Testimony,* 2001 Pontifical Council of Health-care Workers, Rome, Italy.
5. Annalena Tonelli, April 28, 1971, in *Lettere dal Kenya.*
6. Annalena Tonelli, May 12, 1971, in *Lettere dal Kenya.*
7. Annalena Tonelli, *Vatican Testimony.*
8. Lindsay Isaac, "Scurvy. TB. Scarlet Fever. They're all back." CNN, December 23, 2015.
9. Ethnomed, Somali Tuberculosis Cultural Profile.
10. Annalena Tonelli to Andrea Saletti, 1970, in *Lettere dal Kenya.*
11. Annalena Tonelli to Guido Tonelli, September 23, 1972, in *Lettere dal Kenya.*
12. Annalena Tonelli, January 23, 1973, in *Lettere dal Kenya.*
13. Annalena Tonelli, a transcript of a recorded message to the Comitato, in *Lettere dal Kenya.*
14. Annalena Tonelli, March 27, 1972, in *Lettere dal Kenya.*
15. Annalena Tonelli, October 31, 1973, in *Lettere dal Kenya.*

6. The Cutting

1. Annalena Tonelli, August 26, 1969, in *Lettere dal Kenya.*
2. Samuel Zwemer, "The Glory of the Impossible," in *Perspectives on the World Christian Movement,* Ralph Winter and Stephen Hawthorne (Pasadena: William Carey Library, 1981), 259.
3. McMillen, *Discovering Tuberculosis,* 136.
4. Paul Farmer, *Pathologies of Power* (Berkeley: University of California Press, 2004), 165.
5. Paul Farmer, *Infections and Inequalities* (Berkeley: University of California Press, 2001), 187.
6. Gazit, *The Forgotten Plague.*

7. The Bismallah Manyatta

1. Ministry of Health report, "TB in Wajir," typed document from Bruno Tonelli.
2. Annalena Tonelli, *Vatican Testimony.*
3. "TB in Wajir" report.
4. Annalena Tonelli, *Vatican Testimony.*
5. "TB in Wajir" report.
6. Abdikarim Sheik-Mohamed, Johan P. Velema, "Where health care has no access: the nomadic populations of sub-Saharan Africa," Abstract, 2002.
7. "TB in Wajir" report and other documents from Bruno Tonelli.
8. Ivan Oransky, "Annalena Tonelli," *The Lancet* 362, no. 9399 December 6, 2003, 1943.

9.   Annalena Tonelli, May 28, 1977, in *Lettere dal Kenya*.
10. Annalena Tonelli, in *Lettere dal Kenya*.
11. Tracy Kidder, *Mountains Beyond Mountains* (New York: Random House, 2009), 100.
12. Mark Klemper, "Conversation with Tracy Kidder," *Huffington Post*, March 16, 2008.
13. Annalena Tonelli, October 29, 1978, in *Lettere dal Kenya*.
14. Gianni Saporetti, "Interview with Maria Teresa Battistini, Enza Laporta, Bruno Tonelli," *Una Citta*, November 2003.
15. Annalena Tonelli, January 15, 1980, in *Lettere dal Kenya*.
16. Annalena Tonelli, May 13, 1971, in *Lettere dal Kenya*.
17. Saporetti, "Interview with Maria Teresa Battistini, Enza Laporta, Bruno Tonelli."
18. Annalena Tonelli, October 29, 1978, in *Lettere dal Kenya*.
19. Ministry of Health, "Wajir Tuberculosis Treatment Project," one year report, typed document from Bruno Tonelli.
20. Annalena Tonelli to Maria Teresa, September 30, 1982, in *Lettere dal Kenya*.

8. Retreat

1.   Annalena Tonelli to Maria Teresa, September 30, 1982, in *Lettere dal Kenya*.
2.   Annalena Tonelli, *Vatican Testimony*.
3.   Annalena Tonelli to Teresina Tonelli, December 23, 1983, in *Lettere dal Kenya*.
4.   Name changed from Mohamed to avoid confusion.
5.   Annalena Tonelli, January 13, 1979, in *Lettere dal Kenya*.
6.   Salah Abdi Sheikh, *Blood on the Runway: The Wagalla Massacre of 1984* (Nairobi: Northern Publishing House, 2007), 141.
7.   Annalena Tonelli, January 2, 1984, in *Lettere dal Kenya*.
8.   Annalena Tonelli, March 1980, in *Lettere dal Kenya*.
9.   Annalena Tonelli, November 5, 1982, in *Lettere dal Kenya*.
10. Annalena Tonelli, November 28, 1980, in *Lettere dal Kenya*.
11. The Final Report of the Truth, Justice, and Reconciliation Commission of Kenya, Volume IV, 2013, page 258.

9. Wagalla

1.   Papers of Nancy Caroline, 1905–2007. Schlesinger Library, Radcliffe Institute. Subseries C, Africa (#42.8-45.10), Harvard Library, Boston, MA, USA.
2.   Papers of Nancy Caroline, photos 1795–7.
3.   Judy Kibinge, director, *Scarred, Anatomy of a Massacre*, Documentary, (Kenya: 2015).
4.   Papers of Nancy Caroline.
5.   Papers of Nancy Caroline.
6.   Papers of Nancy Caroline.
7.   Papers of Nancy Caroline.
8.   Papers of Nancy Caroline.

9. Report of the Truth, Justice, and Reconciliation Commission, Volume IV, 2013.
10. Papers of Nancy Caroline.
11. Annalena Tonelli, September 20, 1984, in *Lettere dal Kenya*.
12. Papers of Nancy Caroline.
13. Annalena Tonelli, February 29, 1984, in *Lettere dal Kenya*.
14. Annalena Tonelli to Leo White, Bishop of Garissa, March 12, 1984, in *Lettere dal Kenya*.
15. Annalena Tonelli to Maria Teresa, June 25, 1984, in *Lettere dal Kenya*.
16. Papers of Nancy Caroline.
17. Annalena Tonelli, January 24, 1985, in *Lettere dal Kenya*.

10. Beledweyne

1. Luca Vitali, *La compassione nell'esistenza di Annalena Tonelli* (Comitato per la Lotta contro la Fame nel Mondo, 2015), 37.
2. Annalena Tonelli to Maria Teresa, April 7, 1987, in *Lettere dal Somalia*, B. Tonelli, E. Laporta, M. Battistini (Bologna: EBD, 2016).
3. Annalena Tonelli to Teresina Tonelli, June 15, 1990, in *Lettere dal Somalia*.
4. Annalena Tonelli to Bruno Tonelli and Enza Laporta, April 14, 1987, in *Lettere dal Somalia*.
5. Annalena Tonelli to Bruno Tonelli, June 5, 1987, in *Lettere dal Somalia*.
6. Annalena Tonelli, *Vatican Testimony*.
7. Annalena Tonelli to Teresina Tonelli, December 25, 1988, in *Lettere dal Somalia*.
8. Michael Maren, *The Road to Hell: The Ravaging Effects of Foreign Aid and International Charity* (New York: Free Press, 2002).
9. Teju Cole, "The White Savior Industrial Complex," *Atlantic*, March 21, 2012.
10. Annalena Tonelli, August 4, 1987, in *Lettere dal Somalia*.
11. Annalena Tonelli to Maria Teresa, June 12, 1987, in *Lettere dal Somalia*.

11. Hostage

1. Annalena Tonelli to Teresina Tonelli, June 15, 1990, in *Lettere dal Somalia*.
2. Annalena Tonelli to Teresina Tonelli, July 1990, in *Lettere dal Somalia*.

12. Mogadishu

1. Annalena Tonelli to Teresina Tonelli, October 24, 1990, in *Lettere dal Somalia*.
2. Scott Peterson, *Me Against My Brother: At War in Somalia, Sudan, and Rwanda* (New York: Rutledge, 2001), 22.
3. Mary Harper, *Getting Somalia Wrong?: Faith, War and Hope in a Shattered State* (London: Zed Books, 2012).
4. Annalena Tonelli to "Beloved," May 21, 1991, in *Lettere dal Somalia*.
5. Peterson, *Me Against My Brother*, 44.
6. Peterson, *Me Against My Brother*, xix.
7. Annalena Tonelli to Teresina Tonelli, April 11, 1991, in *Lettere dal Somalia*.
8. Annalena Tonelli to Teresina Tonelli, May 1, 1991, in *Lettere dal Somalia*.

9.   Mario Neri, *Lorenzo: Lettera a mio figlio* (Iacobelli, 2011).
10. Annalena Tonelli to Maria Teresa, April 11, 1991, in *Lettere dal Somalia*.
11. Peterson, *Me Against My Brother*, 20.
12. Peterson, *Me Against My Brother*, 39.
13. Annalena Tonelli to Teresina Tonelli, September 14, 1991, in *Lettere dal Somalia*.

13. Merka

1.   Suzanne M. Marks et al., "Treatment Practices, Outcomes, and Costs of Multidrug-Resistant and Extensively Drug-Resistant Tuberculosis, United States, 2005–2007," *Emerging Infectious Diseases* 20, no. 5 (May 2014): 812–821.
2.   Annalena Tonelli to Teresina Tonelli, October 24, 1990, in *Lettere dal Somalia*.
3.   David Brown, "A Breath of Fresh Air," *Washington Post*, February 24, 1993.
4.   Annalena Tonelli to Teresina Tonelli, October 17, 1992, in *Lettere dal Somalia*.
5.   Rudi Coninx, "Tuberculosis in Complex Emergencies," September 2007.
6.   Brown, "A Breath of Fresh Air."
7.   Neri, *Lorenzo*.
8.   Annalena Tonelli to Joe Morrissey, February 23, 1992, in *Lettere dal Somalia*.
9.   Mission to Somalia, transcript of President George H. W. Bush's speech, 1992, Associated Press.
10. Vitali, *La compassione nell'esistenza di Annalena Tonelli*, 2015.
11. Peterson, *Me Against My Brother*, 60.
12. Annalena Tonelli, January 1, 1993, in *Lettere dal Somalia*.
13. Peterson, *Me Against My Brother*, 69.
14. Brown, "A Breath of Fresh Air."

14. Complex Emergencies

1.   Greg Myre, "Italian Miracle Worker In Land Where Hope Seems Lost," *Associated Press*, September 2, 1992.
2.   Annalena Tonelli, December 26, 1991, in *Lettere dal Somalia*.
3.   Annalena Tonelli to Halima, June 6, 1992, in *Lettere dal Somalia*.
4.   Annalena Tonelli to Joe Morrissey, August 18, 1992, in *Lettere dal Somalia*.
5.   Sam Kiley, "Treatment fails to help starving Somali children," *Times (UK)*, May 18, 1992.
6.   David Brown, "The Healing Heart of Annalena Tonelli," *Washington Post*, October 8, 2003.
7.   Annalena Tonelli to Teresina Tonelli, February 24, 1993, in *Lettere dal Somalia*.
8.   Charles Geshekter, "Death of Somalia," in *Mending Rips in the Sky*, Hussein M. Adam and Richard Ford (Lawrenceville, NJ: Red Sea Press, 1997).
9.   Neri, *Lorenzo*.

10. Annalena Tonelli, October 31, 1995, in *Lettere dal Somalia*.

11. Annalena Tonelli, *Vatican Testimony*.

12. Saporetti, "Interview with Maria Teresa Battistini, Enza Laporta, Bruno Tonelli."

15. Borama

1. Annalena Tonelli, letter to SAGB TB Working Group, 1999.

2. 2003 July TB Report, document shown to the author by Bishop Giorgio.

3. Annalena Tonelli, *Vatican Testimony*.

4. Annalena Tonelli, March 26, 1996 to Bruno Tonelli, in *Lettere dal Somaliland*, B. Tonelli, E. Laporta, M. Battistini (Bologna: EBD, 2018).

5. Annalena Tonelli to Andrea Saletti, April 27, 1997, in *Lettere dal Somaliland*.

6. Maggie Black, "The time has come to disarm. Lay down your weapons." *Guardian*, January 25, 2004.

7. FGM training speech, typed notes from Bruno Tonelli.

8. Black, "The time has come to disarm."

16. The Nansen Award

1. "Annalena: A Christian of Tomorrow," compiled speeches from Annalena's friends and family (unpublished manuscript).

2. Anna Pozzi, "Annalena: un silenzio che parla," *Mondo e Missione,* November 2003.

3. Annalena Tonelli, November 2, 2002, in *Lettere dal Somaliland*.

4. Maria Teresa Battistini speech at The Parish of St. Stefano, Paterno, 2009.

5. Maria Teresa Battistini speech at The Parish of St. Stefano, Paterno, 2009.

17. Legacy

1. Vivian Tan, "Jolie releases online journal on mission to Russian Federation," UNHCR, January 26, 2004.

2. Kitty McKinsey and Laura Boldrini, "Mourners remember Dr. Tonelli, pledge to continue her work," UNHCR, October 14, 2003.

Other Titles from Plough

The 21: A Journey into the Land of Coptic Martyrs
Martin Mosebach
Behind an ISIS beheading video lies the untold story of the
men in orange and the faith community that formed them.

**From Red Earth: A Rwandan Story of
Healing and Forgiveness**
Denise Uwimana
A hundred days of carnage, twenty-five years of rebirth.

The Reckless Way of Love: Notes on Following Jesus
Dorothy Day
How do you follow Jesus without burning out?

**The Last Christians: Stories of Persecution, Flight,
and Resilience in the Middle East**
Andreas Knapp
A Westerner's travels among the persecuted and displaced
Christian remnant in Iraq and Syria.

**Bearing Witness: Stories of Martyrdom and
Costly Discipleship**
Charles E. Moore and Timothy J. Keiderling
Stories of Christian martyrs from around the world and
through the ages.

Plough Publishing House
PO BOX 398, Walden, NY 12586, USA
Robertsbridge, East Sussex TN32 5DR, UK
4188 Gwydir Highway, Elsmore, NSW 2360, Australia
845-572-3455 • info@plough.com • *www.plough.com*